Simply Well

Managing Type 2 Diabetes:
A Basic Guide to Wellness

Table of Contents

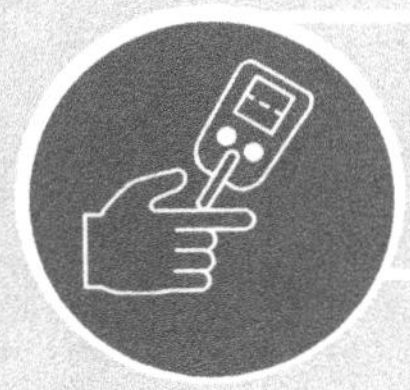

Dear Valued Reader,

Thank you for embarking on this journey with "Simply Well: Managing Type 2 Diabetes." Our purpose is simple yet profound – to equip you with the knowledge and encouragement needed for the effective and easy management of Type 2 Diabetes.

This book is crafted in a format that values your time, ensuring a quick and accessible read. The extra-large print aims to eliminate any strain on your eyes, prioritizing your comfort and ease of understanding.

As a small publishing house, your feedback is invaluable. If you find value in these pages, we kindly ask you to share your thoughts with a review. Your insights not only shape our future endeavors but also contribute to the well-being of others on a similar path.

Wishing you health, happiness, and a fulfilling journey through these pages.

Warm regards,
Shaffer Publishing

Simply Well

Managing Type 2 Diabetes:
A Basic Guide to Wellness

Welcome to the pages of Simply Well Managing Type 2 Diabetes: A Basic Guide to Wellness " As you embark on this journey, it is important to note that the information provided within these chapters is not a substitute for professional medical advice. I am not a medical professional, and this book is crafted for educational purposes only.

The Purpose of This Book:
The goal of this book is to empower individuals with type 2 diabetes by providing comprehensive information on key elements that contribute to a healthier life. From nutrition and exercise to the importance of sunlight, fresh water, breath work, and mental well-being, each chapter delves into crucial aspects of holistic health.

Disclaimer:
In navigating the vast landscape of managing type 2 diabetes, it is crucial to consult with your healthcare provider for personalized guidance. The content within this book is based on extensive research, personal experiences, and a commitment to fostering awareness about the multifaceted aspects of living with type 2 diabetes.

Type 2 diabetes is a complex condition that requires a holistic approach to wellness. This book aims to complement the advice and care provided by healthcare professionals, offering insights into various facets of a healthy lifestyle. It is not a replacement for the expertise of your medical team, who can provide tailored recommendations based on your unique health profile.

Navigating the Chapters:
Throughout the chapters, you will find practical advice, research-backed insights, and suggested lifestyle adjustments. It is important to approach this information with an open mind, recognizing that every person's journey with type 2 diabetes is unique. What works well for one individual may require adaptation for another.

Your Primary Resource:
Your healthcare provider remains your primary resource for managing type 2 diabetes. Before making significant changes to your diet, exercise routine, or treatment plan, consult with your healthcare team to ensure alignment with your specific health needs and goals.

Celebrating Progress:
As you engage with the content in this book, consider keeping a journal to track your progress and reflect on how these insights integrate into your daily life. Small victories matter, and this book is designed to support you on your path to a healthier and more fulfilling life.

Now, let's embark on the exploration of managing type 2 diabetes, embracing the knowledge within these pages as a supplement to the guidance provided by your healthcare team.

Chapter One

Understanding the Prevalence and Impact of Type 2 Diabetes

Type 2 diabetes has emerged as a widespread health concern, affecting millions of individuals globally. The prevalence of this condition has surged in recent years, reaching epidemic proportions. This chapter aims to shed light on the prevalence of type 2 diabetes and its profound impact on the lives of those living with the condition.

According to the International Diabetes Federation (IDF) and the World Health Organization (WHO), it was estimated that over 460 million adults (20-79 years old) were living with diabetes worldwide in 2019. Type 2 diabetes accounts for the majority of diabetes cases, representing around 90-95% of all diagnosed cases.

Trends and Projections:
Type 2 diabetes has been on the rise globally, and this trend is expected to continue. Factors such as urbanization, sedentary lifestyles, and dietary changes contribute to the increasing incidence of type 2 diabetes. Projections suggest that by the year 2045, the number of adults with diabetes could rise to over 700 million globally if current trends persist.

Impact on Healthcare Systems:
The growing prevalence of type 2 diabetes places a significant burden on healthcare systems worldwide. The condition is associated with various complications, including cardiovascular diseases, kidney problems, and neuropathy, leading to increased healthcare costs and resource utilization.

My awareness of Type 2 Diabetes traces back to my childhood, where poignant memories were etched during visits to a Veteran's Hospital with my family. It was there that I first encountered the impact of Diabetes on my aging uncle. In those days, people commonly referred to it as "Sugar Diabetes," a term that sparked my curiosity as a little girl. The paradox of something as enjoyable as sugar being associated with health issues lingered in my mind.

As the years passed, the specter of Type 2 Diabetes cast its shadow on many fronts, affecting friends and cherished family members, including my beloved grandmother. Witnessing their struggles fueled my determination to make a positive impact. Intrigued by the transformative potential of a healthy lifestyle and diet for individuals with Type 2 Diabetes, I embarked on a journey of research and culinary exploration.

The culmination of this endeavor was the creation of "Diabetic Delights Large Print," a cookbook designed specifically for those managing diabetes. The positive response, particularly on the associated Facebook page, revealed a broader need for accessible and concise information on the subject. Many expressed the desire for straightforward, quick insights that could be easily incorporated into their lives.

Motivated by this feedback, I felt a calling to delve deeper. Recognizing the importance of time and simplicity in our fast-paced lives, I set out to research and write a comprehensive yet succinct large print book. My aim was to distill valuable information into a format that wouldn't demand an extensive time commitment to read, offering a source of encouragement and empowerment for individuals navigating the complexities of Type 2 Diabetes.

This book seeks to bridge the gap between awareness and action, providing easily digestible insights that empower those with Type 2 Diabetes to make informed choices on their journey toward better health. Through this endeavor, my hope is to inspire positive change, one reader at a time.

What is Type 2 Diabetes? In understanding Type 2 Diabetes, it's essential to grasp the fundamental definition and basics that underlie this complex condition. This section aims to provide readers with a clear foundation, demystifying the nature of Type 2 Diabetes.

Type 2 Diabetes is a chronic metabolic disorder characterized by the body's inability to effectively use insulin, a hormone that regulates blood sugar (glucose). Unlike Type 1 Diabetes, where the body doesn't produce insulin, individuals with Type 2 Diabetes often produce insulin, but their cells resist its effects, leading to elevated blood sugar levels.

Basics of Insulin Resistance:
Insulin, a hormone produced by the pancreas, plays a crucial role in regulating blood sugar levels. Its primary function is to facilitate the absorption of glucose into cells for energy utilization. In a healthy body, this process operates smoothly. However, in individuals with Type 2 Diabetes, the concept of insulin resistance comes into play, disrupting this delicate balance.

 To understand this better Let's delve into the normal function of insulin.

After we consume food, especially carbohydrates, the digestive system breaks down these carbohydrates into glucose, a form of sugar. In response to the rise in blood glucose levels after a meal, the pancreas releases insulin into the bloodstream.

Insulin acts like a key that unlocks the doors of cells, particularly muscle, fat, and liver cells. The cell membranes have insulin receptors, which are proteins that respond to the presence of insulin.

When insulin binds to these receptors, it triggers a series of intracellular events that facilitate the uptake of glucose into the cells. This process is essential for providing cells with the energy they need for various functions, including muscle contraction, energy storage, and maintaining metabolic balance.

Once inside the cells, glucose can be used immediately for energy or converted into glycogen for storage in the liver and muscles.

This storage form of glucose can be later converted back into glucose when energy is needed.

Insulin also plays a role in inhibiting the release of glucose from the liver into the bloodstream. This helps regulate blood sugar levels, preventing them from becoming too high.

Insulin is not only involved in glucose metabolism but also influences the metabolism of lipids (fats) and proteins. It promotes the storage of fats in fat cells and supports protein synthesis. Insulin acts as a key player in the intricate system that regulates glucose metabolism. Its normal function ensures that cells receive the necessary energy from glucose, helps maintain blood sugar levels within a narrow range, and plays a role in overall metabolic balance. Understanding this is crucial for appreciating how disruptions, such as insulin resistance, can lead to imbalances and contribute to conditions like Type 2 Diabetes.

Cell Resistance: Understanding Insulin Resistance

Insulin resistance is a key feature in the development and progression of Type 2 Diabetes. It involves a scenario where cells in the body, especially muscle, fat, and liver cells, become less responsive to the signals of insulin. Despite the pancreas producing insulin, the cells exhibit resistance, hindering the normal process of glucose absorption.

Factors Contributing to Insulin Resistance:
Genetic Predisposition: Some individuals may have a genetic predisposition to reduced insulin sensitivity. Genetic factors can influence the function of insulin receptors and the efficiency of intracellular processes.

Lifestyle Factors: Poor lifestyle choices, including a diet high in processed sugars and fats, sedentary behavior, and obesity, can contribute to the development of insulin resistance. Excess fat, particularly visceral fat around the abdomen, is closely linked to increased insulin resistance.

Insulin Signaling Pathway Disruptions:
Normal Insulin Signaling: In a healthy individual, when insulin binds to its receptors on the cell membrane, it initiates a signaling pathway inside the cell. This pathway facilitates the movement of glucose transporters to the cell surface, allowing glucose to enter the cell.

Insulin Resistance Disruptions: In insulin resistance, the normal signaling pathway is disrupted. The insulin receptors may become less sensitive or downregulated, impairing the cell's ability to respond to insulin effectively.

Impaired Glucose Uptake:
Muscle Cells: Insulin resistance in muscle cells means that these cells are less efficient at taking up glucose, especially after meals. This results in elevated blood glucose levels.

Fat Cells: Adipose tissue (fat cells) also experiences reduced responsiveness to insulin, leading to impaired storage of excess glucose as fat. This contributes to higher circulating levels of free fatty acids.

Liver Cells: In the liver, insulin resistance disrupts the normal inhibition of glucose production. The liver releases more glucose into the bloodstream, further contributing to elevated blood sugar levels.

Hyperinsulinemia and Pancreatic Compensation:
Increased Insulin Production:* To compensate for the resistance, the pancreas increases insulin production, resulting in elevated insulin levels in the bloodstream (hyperinsulinemia).

Progressive Strain on the Pancreas: Over time, the pancreas may struggle to maintain this heightened production, leading to a gradual decline in insulin secretion. This progressive strain on the pancreas contributes to the advancement of Type 2 Diabetes.

Consequences and Health Implications:
Elevated Blood Sugar Levels: The primary consequence of insulin resistance is elevated blood sugar levels, as cells are unable to efficiently absorb glucose.

Contributing to Complications: Prolonged insulin resistance contributes to the development of complications associated with Type 2 Diabetes, such as cardiovascular issues, kidney disease, and nerve damage.

Understanding insulin resistance is crucial for developing effective strategies for managing and preventing Type 2 Diabetes. Lifestyle modifications, including a balanced diet, regular physical activity, and weight management, play pivotal roles in addressing insulin resistance and promoting overall health.

Nervous System:
Peripheral Neuropathy: Elevated blood sugar levels can cause damage to nerves, particularly in the extremities. Peripheral neuropathy can result in pain, tingling, and numbness in the hands and feet.

Autonomic Neuropathy: Diabetes can affect the autonomic nervous system, leading to issues with digestion, blood pressure regulation, and other involuntary functions.

Increased Risk of Nerve Damage: Long-term uncontrolled diabetes increases the risk of severe nerve damage, impacting overall neurological function.

Eyes:
Diabetic Retinopathy: Elevated blood sugar can damage the blood vessels in the eyes, leading to diabetic retinopathy. This condition is a leading cause of vision loss in individuals with diabetes.

Increased Risk of Cataracts and Glaucoma: Diabetes also increases the risk of developing cataracts and glaucoma.

Skin:
Increased Susceptibility to Infections: Elevated blood sugar levels may compromise the immune system, making individuals with diabetes more susceptible to skin infections.
Delayed Wound Healing: Diabetes can impair the body's ability to heal wounds, leading to delayed recovery from injuries.

Impact on the Body: Elevated Blood Sugar and Long-Term Complications

Elevated blood sugar levels, a hallmark of Type 2 Diabetes, can have profound effects on multiple organs and systems in the body. Understanding these impacts is crucial for comprehending the long-term complications associated with uncontrolled diabetes.

Cardiovascular System:

Atherosclerosis- Prolonged high blood sugar can contribute to the development of atherosclerosis, a condition where arteries become narrowed and hardened due to the accumulation of plaque. This increases the risk of heart disease, heart attacks, and strokes.

Hypertension: Diabetes can lead to high blood pressure, further straining the cardiovascular system and increasing the risk of heart-related complications.

Increased Risk of Blood Vessel Damage: Elevated glucose levels can damage blood vessels, leading to poor circulation and potential complications in various organs.

Kidneys:

Diabetic Nephropathy: Persistent high blood sugar can damage the kidneys, leading to diabetic nephropathy. This condition involves the gradual loss of kidney function and an increased risk of kidney failure.

Increased Protein in Urine: Damaged kidneys may allow proteins to leak into the urine, a sign of impaired kidney function.

Reproductive System:
Fertility Issues: Uncontrolled diabetes can contribute to fertility issues in both men and women.
Complications during Pregnancy: Women with diabetes may face complications during pregnancy, including a higher risk of gestational diabetes and birth complications.

Gastrointestinal System:
Digestive Issues: Diabetes can affect the nerves that control digestion, leading to issues such as gastroparesis, a condition where the stomach takes longer to empty.

Elevated blood sugar levels, when left uncontrolled, can have far-reaching consequences on various organs and systems. The potential long-term complications underscore the importance of proactive diabetes management, emphasizing lifestyle modifications, regular monitoring, and collaboration with healthcare professionals to minimize these risks.

Distinction from Type 1 Diabetes: Understanding the Differences

It's crucial to distinguish between Type 1 and Type 2 Diabetes, as they are distinct conditions with different causes, characteristics, and management approaches. While both involve issues with insulin, they have key differences that shape their respective nature.

Causes:
Type 1 Diabetes: This form is primarily an autoimmune condition where the immune system mistakenly attacks and destroys the insulin-producing beta cells in the pancreas. Individuals with **Type 1 Diabetes** typically require lifelong insulin injections since their bodies produce little to no insulin.
Type 2 Diabetes: The primary factors contributing to Type 2 Diabetes are insulin resistance and relative insulin deficiency. Insulin resistance means cells are less responsive to insulin, and over time, the pancreas may struggle to produce enough insulin to meet the body's needs.

Age of Onset:
Type 1 Diabetes: Often diagnosed in childhood or adolescence, although it can occur at any age.
Type 2 Diabetes: Typically develops in adulthood, but with the rise in childhood obesity, there is an increasing incidence of Type 2 Diabetes in younger individuals.

Autoimmune Component:
Type 1 Diabetes: Involves an autoimmune response, where the immune system mistakenly attacks and destroys insulin-producing beta cells in the pancreas.
Type 2 Diabetes: While inflammation may play a role, there is no autoimmune component. The primary issue is insulin resistance and a decline in insulin production over time.

Insulin Production:
Type 1 Diabetes: Individuals with Type 1 Diabetes produce little to no insulin and require external insulin sources for survival.
Type 2 Diabetes: Initially, the pancreas produces insulin, but cells become resistant to its effects. Over time, insulin production may decline, leading to relative insulin deficiency.

Body Weight:
Type 1 Diabetes: Not linked to body weight or lifestyle factors.
Type 2 Diabetes: Often associated with obesity and sedentary lifestyle, although genetic factors also play a role.

Management Approaches:
Type 1 Diabetes: Requires insulin therapy from the time of diagnosis. Various types of insulin (short-acting, long-acting) are used to mimic the body's natural insulin production.
Type 2 Diabetes: Management typically begins with lifestyle modifications, including diet and exercise. Medications may be prescribed, and in some cases, insulin therapy may be needed. Lifestyle changes play a crucial role in managing and preventing complications.

Risk Factors:

Type 1 Diabetes: Family history and genetic predisposition are risk factors. No direct association with lifestyle choices.

Type 2 Diabetes: Risk factors include family history, obesity, sedentary lifestyle, age, and certain ethnic backgrounds.

In summary, while both Type 1 and Type 2 Diabetes involve issues with insulin, their causes, age of onset, autoimmune involvement, and management approaches are distinct. Recognizing these differences is essential for accurate diagnosis and tailoring effective treatment plans for individuals with diabetes.

Diagnostic Criteria for Type 2 Diabetes: Early Detection and Importance

Timely and accurate diagnosis of Type 2 Diabetes is crucial for initiating appropriate management strategies and minimizing the risk of complications. The diagnostic criteria involve assessing blood glucose levels through specific tests. Here's an introduction to the diagnostic criteria and the significance of early detection:

Fasting Plasma Glucose Test (FPG):
Criteria: A fasting plasma glucose test measures blood sugar levels after an overnight fast. A diagnosis of Type 2 Diabetes is considered if the fasting glucose level is equal to or exceeds 126 milligrams per deciliter (mg/dL) on two separate occasions.

Oral Glucose Tolerance Test (OGTT):
Criteria: The OGTT involves fasting overnight and then consuming a beverage with a standardized amount of glucose. Blood sugar levels are tested two hours after consuming the glucose solution. A diagnosis of Type 2 Diabetes is made if the blood glucose level is equal to or exceeds 200 mg/dL.

Hemoglobin A1c Test:
Criteria: The hemoglobin A1c test measures the average blood sugar levels over the past two to three months. A diagnosis of Type 2 Diabetes is considered if the A1c level is 6.5% or higher.

Importance of Early Detection and Diagnosis:

Preventing Complications:
Early detection allows for the prompt initiation of management strategies, reducing the risk of complications associated with uncontrolled diabetes. Complications include cardiovascular diseases, kidney problems, nerve damage, and vision impairment.

Lifestyle Modifications:
An early diagnosis provides individuals with the opportunity to make lifestyle modifications that can positively impact blood sugar levels. This includes adopting a healthy diet, engaging in regular physical activity, and managing body weight.

Medication and Insulin Therapy:
In some cases, early diagnosis may lead to the timely initiation of medications or insulin therapy, helping to regulate blood glucose levels and prevent further deterioration of pancreatic function.

Patient Education:
Early diagnosis allows for comprehensive patient education on diabetes management. Individuals can learn about monitoring blood sugar levels, recognizing symptoms of hyperglycemia or hypoglycemia, and making informed choices about diet and exercise

Improved Quality of Life:
Timely intervention and management contribute to an improved quality of life for individuals with Type 2 Diabetes. Addressing the condition early can mitigate its impact on daily activities and overall well-being.

Public Health Impact:
Early detection on a broader scale has public health implications, as it enables healthcare providers to implement preventive measures and educational campaigns to address the rising incidence of Type 2 Diabetes.

Early detection and diagnosis of Type 2 Diabetes are essential components of effective diabetes care. By identifying the condition early, healthcare professionals and individuals can work collaboratively to implement strategies that enhance overall health and minimize the risk of complications associated with uncontrolled diabetes. Regular screenings, especially for individuals with risk factors, play a key role in achieving these goals.

Receiving a diagnosis of Type 2 Diabetes can be an overwhelming experience for patients. While this chapter delves into potential serious situations associated with the condition, its purpose is to create awareness about the gravity of the matter. The intent of this book is to inspire readers to actively participate in activities that enhance their overall health. Throughout the chapters, we will explore dietary and lifestyle changes that have proven beneficial for numerous individuals. Here are some examples of the positive impact these changes have had on people's lives:

John was diagnosed with Type 2 Diabetes after experiencing symptoms like increased thirst and frequent urination. With guidance from healthcare professionals, John embraced a comprehensive approach. He adopted a balanced diet, engaged in regular exercise, and attended diabetes education programs. Over time, John lost weight, improved his blood sugar control, and reduced his reliance on medication. His commitment to a healthy lifestyle contributed to a significant improvement in his overall well-being.

Maria, a middle-aged woman, learned about her Type 2 Diabetes diagnosis during a routine check-up. Motivated to make positive changes, Maria revamped her lifestyle. She incorporated nutrient-dense foods, monitored portion sizes, and started a daily exercise routine, including walking and yoga. Maria not only achieved better blood sugar control but also experienced increased energy levels and improved mood. Her commitment to ongoing self-care contributed to her sustained success in managing diabetes.

Tom had a family history of Type 2 Diabetes and was diagnosed during a health screening.
Tom's healthcare team prescribed medication to manage his blood sugar levels. Additionally, he diligently monitored his blood glucose regularly and attended regular follow-ups with his healthcare provider.
Through a combination of medication adherence and vigilant monitoring, Tom achieved stable blood sugar levels. His proactive approach, coupled with ongoing support, allowed him to lead a fulfilling life while effectively managing his diabetes.

Sophie was diagnosed with Type 2 Diabetes and felt overwhelmed by the lifestyle changes required. Recognizing the importance of emotional well-being, Sophie sought support from family, friends, and a diabetes support group. She attended counseling sessions to address the emotional aspects of living with a chronic condition.
Sophie found strength in her support network, enabling her to cope with the challenges of diabetes. With a holistic approach that addressed both physical and emotional aspects, she successfully managed her condition and improved her overall quality of life.

Chapter Two

The Value of Food

Welcome to Chapter 2, where we delve into the vital role that food plays in managing Type 2 Diabetes. Nutrition is not just a daily necessity but a powerful tool that can significantly influence your health journey. In this chapter, we will explore the profound impact that food choices can have on managing and even reversing Type 2 Diabetes.

The Power of Nutrition in Managing Type 2 Diabetes
Receiving a diagnosis of Type 2 Diabetes can feel like navigating uncharted territory, but the choices you make in your daily diet can be transformative. Nutrition is the cornerstone of diabetes management, and this chapter is dedicated to unraveling the importance of what you eat and its potential to shape your health outcomes.

In managing Type 2 Diabetes, nutrition takes center stage as a key player in achieving optimal health. It goes beyond counting calories; it involves making informed and intentional choices that nourish your body and support your well-being. This chapter aims to shed light on the profound impact that nutrition can have on your journey towards a healthier and more balanced life.

Food is not merely sustenance; it is a powerful tool that can either exacerbate or alleviate the effects of Type 2 Diabetes. Through mindful food choices, you have the ability to regulate blood sugar levels, improve energy levels, and enhance overall vitality. This chapter emphasizes the role of food as a dynamic and integral part of your health toolkit.

Navigating the Chapter:
As we navigate this chapter, we will explore the nutritional needs specific to individuals with Type 2 Diabetes. We'll uncover the potential risks associated with unhealthy food choices and, more importantly, unveil the positive impact that a healthy diet can have on managing and even preventing the progression of this condition.

Get ready to embark on a journey of discovery, where we'll unravel the secrets of nourishing your body, making informed dietary decisions, and embracing the transformative power of food in the realm of Type 2 Diabetes management. It's time to see food not just as sustenance but as a valuable ally on your path to improved health.

Understanding Nutritional Needs:
In the realm of Type 2 Diabetes management, a foundational aspect lies in understanding the specific nutritional needs tailored to support your health journey. This exploration delves into the intricacies of nutrition, examining the role of macronutrients and micronutrients in maintaining balance and fostering overall well-being.

Macronutrients: Balancing the Essentials

Carbohydrates:
Carbohydrates, often perceived as the primary culprit in blood sugar fluctuations, play a crucial role in providing energy. In this context, understanding the types of carbohydrates—simple and complex—and their impact on blood sugar levels is pivotal. By choosing complex carbohydrates with fiber, individuals with Type 2 Diabetes can promote sustained energy release and better blood sugar control.

Proteins:
Proteins are the building blocks of life, essential for tissue repair and overall body function. For those managing Type 2 Diabetes, incorporating lean protein sources into their diet is beneficial. These sources include poultry, fish, legumes, and tofu. Balancing protein intake aids in stabilizing blood sugar levels and supporting muscle health.

Fats:
Contrary to common misconceptions, fats are essential for a well-rounded diet. However, the focus should be on healthy fats, such as those found in avocados, nuts, and olive oil. By opting for these sources, individuals with Type 2 Diabetes can promote heart health and overall metabolic balance.

The Power of Vitamins
Vitamins are catalysts for various biochemical processes in the body. Understanding the role of vitamins, such as vitamin D for bone health or vitamin C for immune support, is crucial. For individuals with Type 2 Diabetes, maintaining an adequate supply of vitamins through a diverse and nutrient-rich diet can contribute to overall health.

The Power of Minerals:
Minerals are essential for functions ranging from nerve transmission to maintaining fluid balance. Key minerals like magnesium and potassium play roles in blood sugar regulation. Embracing a diet rich in leafy greens, whole grains, and nuts can help ensure a sufficient intake of these vital minerals.

Tailoring Nutrition for Type 2 Diabetes
In summary, understanding nutritional needs involves a delicate balancing act. By being mindful of the types and amounts of macronutrients consumed and recognizing the importance of micronutrients, individuals with Type 2 Diabetes can craft a diet that not only supports their specific health needs but also empowers them on their journey towards optimal well-being. As we proceed, we'll further explore how these nutritional insights translate into actionable choices for a healthier lifestyle.

Unhealthy Food Choices:
In the landscape of Type 2 Diabetes management, the choices we make regarding our diet wield a profound influence on our well-being. This section is dedicated to unraveling the impact of processed and fast foods—often deemed convenient but laden with potential pitfalls—on blood sugar levels. By exploring the connection between poor food choices and the exacerbation of Type 2 Diabetes, we aim to empower individuals to make informed decisions about what they consume.

The Fast Food Dilemma:
Fast food, characterized by its quick preparation and often enticing flavors, can pose significant challenges for individuals managing Type 2 Diabetes. These offerings are frequently rich in refined carbohydrates, unhealthy fats, and excessive sodium, contributing to rapid spikes in blood sugar levels. The combination of high glycemic index ingredients and processed sugars in fast food can wreak havoc on blood sugar control.

Processed Foods: Culprits in Disguise:
Processed foods, prevalent in modern diets for their convenience, often harbor hidden threats to metabolic health. Loaded with refined sugars, preservatives, and artificial additives, these items can lead to elevated blood sugar levels and hinder insulin sensitivity. The pervasive nature of processed foods in our daily lives makes it crucial to scrutinize labels and be aware of their potential impact on blood glucose.

The Sugar Conundrum:
Added sugars, omnipresent in many processed and fast foods, are linked to increased insulin resistance and heightened inflammation. From sugary beverages to desserts and hidden sugars in sauces, vigilant awareness is essential. Recognizing the detrimental effects of excessive sugar consumption is a pivotal step toward making more health-conscious choices.

The Connection to Type 2 Diabetes:
The correlation between poor food choices and the exacerbation of Type 2 Diabetes is undeniable. Diets rich in processed and fast foods not only contribute to unhealthy weight gain but also escalate insulin resistance. The repetitive cycle of blood sugar spikes and crashes places additional strain on the pancreas, fostering an environment conducive to the progression of Type 2 Diabetes.

Understanding the impact of unhealthy food choices is the first step toward empowerment. By making informed decisions to minimize processed and fast food consumption, individuals with Type 2 Diabetes can regain control over their blood sugar levels. The journey towards improved health involves a mindful approach to nutrition, emphasizing whole, nutrient-dense foods that nourish the body and support long-term well-being.

As we continue to navigate the chapters ahead, we'll explore alternatives and strategies to foster a healthier relationship with food, empowering individuals to make choices that contribute to the effective management of Type 2 Diabetes.

Embarking on a journey of managing Type 2 Diabetes involves recognizing the transformative potential of a healthy diet. In this section, we delve into the profound concept of food as medicine, illuminating how a balanced and nutrient-dense diet can be a cornerstone in positively influencing blood sugar control.

Food as Medicine: A Paradigm Shift:
In the realm of managing diabetes, viewing food as medicine signifies a transformative shift in perspective. Rather than merely being sustenance, each meal becomes an opportunity to nourish the body, support overall health, and actively contribute to diabetes management. This paradigm acknowledges the potent impact that our dietary choices can have on our well-being.

The Balanced Approach:
A healthy diet for individuals with Type 2 Diabetes is rooted in balance—balancing macronutrients, portion sizes, and food choices. Opting for a variety of whole foods, including fruits, vegetables, lean proteins, and whole grains, provides essential nutrients that promote optimal health. This balance is instrumental in regulating blood sugar levels, preventing spikes, and fostering a stable metabolic environment.

Nutrient Density and Blood Sugar Control:
Nutrient-dense foods, rich in vitamins, minerals, and antioxidants, form the bedrock of a healthy diet. These foods not only contribute to overall well-being but also play a pivotal role in blood sugar control. The gradual release of sugars from nutrient-dense sources supports sustained energy levels, minimizing the risk of rapid blood sugar fluctuations.

The Impact on Insulin Sensitivity:
A healthy diet isn't just about what we eat; it's about how our body responds to those choices. A nutrient-dense diet has the potential to enhance insulin sensitivity, allowing cells to effectively utilize insulin for glucose absorption. This shift positively influences blood sugar regulation and reduces the burden on the pancreas, fostering a more resilient metabolic state.

Practical Steps Toward a Healthy Diet:
Incorporating a healthy diet into your lifestyle involves practical steps. It means savoring the vibrant colors of a variety of vegetables, choosing whole grains over refined options, and embracing lean protein sources. It's about mindful eating, savoring each bite, and recognizing the impact of your choices on your overall health.

As we progress through this exploration of the power of a healthy diet, envision it not as a restrictive measure but as an empowering tool in your diabetes management toolkit. Each meal becomes an opportunity to cultivate a positive impact on your health, one that extends beyond blood sugar control to encompass vitality, resilience, and a thriving well-being. The journey ahead is one of discovery, empowerment, and the profound realization that food, when chosen wisely, becomes a catalyst for transformative health.

Nourishing Foods for Type 2 Diabetes:

In the quest for managing Type 2 Diabetes, the significance of nourishing foods cannot be overstated. This section is dedicated to identifying specific foods that offer tangible benefits for individuals with Type 2 Diabetes. By exploring examples of foods rich in fiber, antioxidants, and essential nutrients, we unveil a spectrum of choices that contribute not only to blood sugar control but also to overall well-being.

Fiber-Rich Foods:
Whole Grains: Examples: Quinoa, brown rice, oats, whole wheat. Whole grains are a powerhouse of fiber, supporting digestive health and promoting gradual glucose absorption. They contribute to sustained energy levels and are versatile additions to a balanced diet.

Legumes:
Examples: Lentils, chickpeas, black beans.
Legumes are rich in both fiber and protein, offering a dual benefit. Their slow-digesting nature helps regulate blood sugar levels, making them excellent choices for individuals with Type 2 Diabetes.

Vegetables:
Examples: Broccoli, Brussels sprouts, spinach, kale.
Non-starchy vegetables are low in calories and high in fiber, making them essential components of a diabetes-friendly diet. They provide essential nutrients while contributing to satiety.

Antioxidant-Rich Foods

Berries: Examples: Blueberries, strawberries, raspberries.
Berries are not only delicious but also rich in antioxidants, which play a role in combating oxidative stress associated with diabetes. They're a delightful addition to snacks and desserts.

Dark Leafy Greens:

Examples: Kale, spinach, Swiss chard.
These greens are packed with antioxidants, vitamins, and minerals. Incorporating them into meals supports overall health and contributes to a nutrient-dense diet.

Nuts and Seeds:

Examples: Almonds, walnuts, flaxseeds, chia seeds.
Nuts and seeds are sources of healthy fats, fiber, and antioxidants. Their inclusion in snacks or meals adds a satisfying crunch and nutritional depth.

Essential Nutrients from Whole Foods:

Fatty Fish: Examples: Salmon, mackerel, sardines. Fatty fish provide omega-3 fatty acids, which have anti-inflammatory properties. Including them in the diet supports heart health and complements diabetes management.

Greek Yogurt:

Examples: Plain, non-fat Greek yogurt.
Greek yogurt is a rich source of protein and probiotics. It serves as a satisfying and versatile dairy option, contributing to a balanced and nutrient-rich diet.

Avocado:
Avocado is a nutrient-dense fruit rich in monounsaturated fats, promoting heart health. Its versatility makes it a delightful addition to salads, sandwiches, or as a standalone snack.

Empowering Choices for Balanced Nutrition:
As we explore these nourishing foods, remember that variety is key. Combining different food groups and incorporating a rainbow of colors on your plate ensures a diverse array of nutrients. These choices not only contribute to blood sugar control but also enhance your overall health, creating a foundation for lasting well-being in your journey with Type 2 Diabetes.

Crafting a simple and effective diet plan is a cornerstone in managing Type 2 Diabetes. This section offers a straightforward and practical approach, providing meal ideas, portion control tips, and meal timing suggestions. The goal is to empower individuals with actionable steps that seamlessly integrate into their daily lives, fostering better blood sugar control and overall well-being.

Meal Ideas for a Balanced Diet:

Breakfast:
Option 1 Oatmeal with berries and a handful of nuts.
Option 2: Greek yogurt parfait with sliced fruits and a sprinkle of chia seeds.
Option 3: Avocado Toast Combo
Whole-grain toast (3 stars) + Mashed avocado (4 stars) + Poached eggs
A delicious and nutritious breakfast featuring whole grains, healthy fats from avocado, and protein-packed poached eggs.

Lunch:
Option 1: Grilled chicken or tofu salad with a variety of colorful vegetables.
Option 2:Quinoa bowl with roasted vegetables and a drizzle of olive oil.
Option 3: Quinoa Power Bowl
Quinoa (3 stars) + Roasted sweet potatoes (3 stars) + Black beans (3 stars)
A power-packed lunch combining protein, complex carbs, and fiber for sustained energy.

Snacks:
Option 1: Fresh fruit with a small handful of almonds.
Option 2: Vegetable sticks with hummus.
Option 3: Cottage Cheese Crunch
Cottage cheese (low-fat - 3 stars) + Pineapple chunks (3 stars) +
Handful of walnuts (3 stars)
A satisfying snack with protein-rich cottage cheese, tropical
sweetness, and crunch from walnuts.

Dinner:
Option 1: Baked salmon with steamed broccoli and quinoa.
Option 2: Stir-fried tofu with a medley of colorful bell peppers
and brown rice.
Option 3: Grilled Chicken Salad
Grilled chicken breast (3 stars) + Quinoa (3 stars) + Roasted
vegetables (3 stars)
This meal combines lean protein, whole grains, and colorful
vegetables, offering a balanced and 3-star rated plate.

Portion Control Tips:

Balanced Plates:
Aim to fill half your plate with non-starchy vegetables, one-quarter with lean protein, and one-quarter with whole grains or healthy carbohydrates.

Mindful Eating:
Pay attention to hunger and fullness cues. Eat slowly, savoring each bite, and stop when you feel satisfied.

Smaller, Frequent Meals:
Consider spreading your food intake across smaller, more frequent meals throughout the day to maintain stable blood sugar levels.

Consistent Meal Schedule:
Stick to a consistent meal schedule. Regularity in meal timing can help regulate blood sugar levels and support the effectiveness of insulin.

Consider Pre- and Post-Exercise Meals:
If incorporating physical activity, plan meals around exercise. A balanced snack before and after can provide energy and support recovery.

Evening Snack:
Consider a balanced evening snack if there is a long gap between dinner and bedtime to prevent nighttime hypoglycemia.

Hydration:
Water as the Primary Beverage:
Prioritize water as your main beverage. Staying well-hydrated supports overall health and can help control appetite.

Limit Sugary Drinks:
Minimize or avoid sugary drinks, opting for unsweetened alternatives like herbal tea or infused water. There are several organic fruit teas on the market. Pop a tea bag into a jar of cold water and place in the fridge for a few hours. They make excellent grab and go drinks.

Empowering Lifestyle Integration:
Remember, this plan is a guide, and flexibility is key. Adapt it to suit your preferences and lifestyle. Consult with healthcare professionals or dietitians for personalized advice. By integrating these simple strategies, you can cultivate a sustainable and health-conscious approach to managing Type 2 Diabetes.

The Star Rating System:

Welcome to a unique aspect of our dietary exploration – the Star Rating System. This innovative approach aims to simplify food choices for individuals managing Type 2 Diabetes by assigning star ratings based on their impact on blood sugar levels. This introduction sheds light on the rating criteria, ranging from 1 star (consume in extreme moderation or never) to 4 stars (super healthy for Type 2 Diabetes), empowering you to make informed and health-conscious decisions about the foods you choose.

1 Star ★   (Consume in Extreme Moderation or Never):
  - Foods in this category have a significant impact on blood sugar levels. They often contain high levels of refined sugars, unhealthy fats, or simple carbohydrates that can lead to rapid spikes in glucose. While occasional consumption may be permissible, it is advised to approach these foods with caution and limit intake to prevent adverse effects on blood sugar control.

2 Stars ★★ (Consume Moderately or on Special Occasions):
  - Foods with a 2-star rating are considered moderate in their impact on blood sugar. They may have elements that, if consumed in moderation or on special occasions, can be accommodated within a balanced diet. However, regular and excessive consumption should be approached with mindfulness to prevent fluctuations in blood sugar levels.

3 Stars ★★★ (Nourishing with Little Effect on Blood Sugar):
   - This category includes foods that are considered nourishing and have minimal impact on blood sugar levels. These options are rich in nutrients, fiber, and essential components that support overall health. They can be integrated into the diet more regularly without significant concerns about blood sugar spikes.

4 Stars ★★★★ (Super Healthy for Type 2 Diabetes):
   - The highest rating is reserved for foods that are not only diabetes-friendly but also contribute positively to overall health. These foods are nutrient-dense, low in refined sugars, and promote stable blood sugar levels. Incorporating 4-star foods into your regular diet can be highly beneficial for individuals managing Type 2 Diabetes.

Empowering Your Food Choices:

The Star Rating System is designed to empower you with a quick and easy tool for making health-conscious decisions. As you explore the chapters ahead, you'll encounter specific foods categorized within this system. It's a practical guide to assist you in tailoring your diet to better manage blood sugar levels, promote well-being, and foster a positive relationship with the foods you enjoy. Remember, these ratings are here to support you on your journey toward a healthier and more informed lifestyle.

One Star Foods ★

Here's a list of 50 foods that are rated 1 star in the Star Rating System, indicating that they should be consumed in extreme moderation or avoided for individuals managing Type 2 Diabetes:

1. Soda
2. Candy bars
3. Sugary cereals
4. Frosted pastries
5. Energy drinks
6. Sugary fruit drinks
7. Regular ice cream
8. White bread
9. Sugary yogurt with added toppings
10. Sweetened canned fruits
11. Pancakes with syrup
12. Commercially baked cookies
13. Processed and sugary breakfast bars
14. Regular chocolate
15. Sugary coffee beverages
16. Sweetened granola
17. Flavored popcorn
18. Sugary cocktails
19. Packaged fruit snacks
20. Sugary condiments (e.g., ketchup with added sugar)
21. Candy-coated chocolates
22. Sweetened iced tea
23. Sugary sauces (e.g., teriyaki sauce)
24. Regular doughnuts
25. Sweetened instant oatmeal packets
26. Sugary energy bars
27. Sweetened coffee creamers
28. Deep-fried desserts
29. Fruit-flavored candies
30. Sugary barbecue sauce
31. Sweetened nut butters
32. Regular potato chips
33. Sugary canned soups
34. Sweetened whipped cream
35. Sugary pre-packaged smoothies
36. Sweetened flavored milk
37. Commercially sweetened jams/jellies
38. Candied nuts
39. Sweetened dried fruits
40. Sugary hot chocolate
41. Sugary flavored water
42. Sugary protein bars
43. Regular caramel popcorn
44. Sweetened flavored rice cakes
45. Sugary coleslaw
46. Sugary deli meats with added glazes
47. Sweetened canned vegetables
48. Sugary yogurt drinks
49. Regular fruit pies
50. Sugary frozen fruit treats

Two Star Foods ★★

Here's a list of 50 foods that are rated 2 stars in the Star Rating System, indicating that they can be consumed moderately or on special occasions for individuals managing Type 2 Diabetes:

1. White rice
2. Whole-grain bread (in moderation)
3. Baked beans
4. Bakery muffins
5. Raisins
6. Bran cereal
7. Popcorn with light butter
8. Pineapple juice
9. Low-fat frozen yogurt
10. Honey
11. Fruit-flavored yogurt
12. Instant oatmeal (unsweetened)
13. Dried cranberries
14. Couscous
15. Reduced-fat crackers
16. Whole-grain waffles
17. Baked sweet potato fries
18. Low-fat granola bars
19. Pita bread
20. Light salad dressing
21. Fat-free pretzels
22. Tortilla chips
23. Reduced-fat cream cheese
24. Brown rice cakes
25. Light mayonnaise
26. Balsamic glaze
27. Low-fat cottage cheese
28. Unsweetened applesauce
29. Maple syrup
30. Whole-grain pasta
31. Light whipped topping
32. Reduced-fat peanut butter
33. Whole-grain tortillas
34. Light hot cocoa mix
35. Organic cheese
36. Whole-grain English muffins
37. Soy milk
38. Sugar-free gelatin
39. Salad croutons
40. Caesar dressing
41. Organic refried beans
42. Homemade coleslaw dressing
43. Reduced-fat sour cream
44. Teriyaki sauce
45. Organic mayonnaise
46. Homemade Italian dressing
47. Ranch dressing
48. Organic sausage
49. Bacon (2 Strips)
50. Organic hot dogs

Thee Star Foods ★★★

Here's a list of 50 foods that are rated 3 stars in the Star Rating System, indicating that they are nourishing with little effect on blood sugar for individuals managing Type 2 Diabetes:

11. Citrus Fruits	26. Potatoes
2. Pigeon Peas	27. Ham Steak (non Sugar)
3. Spinach	28. Barley
4. Hot Peppers	29. Whole-grain couscous
5. Clams	30. spaghetti squash
6. Cucumbers	31. Apples
7. Pears	32. Carrots
8. Lettuce	33. Turnips
9. Cauliflower	34. Beets
10. Kidney Beans	35. Brown rice cakes
11. Zucchini	36. Egg Plant
12. Acorn Squash	37. Gouda cheese
13. Lima beans	38. Sharp cheese
14. Crab	39. Mozzarella cheese
15. Cabbage	40. milk
16. Green Beans	41. Dill Pickles
17. Lima Beans	42. Watermelon (1/2 Cup)
18. Pinto Beans	43. Tangerines
19. Grass Fed Butter	44. Oranges
20. Ground Beed Fat Removed	45. Grapes
21. Avocado oil	46. Kiwi
22. Sweet Potatoes	47. Shrimp
23. Vegetarian Cheese	48. Pineapple
24. Lean Pork	49. Unsweetened almond milk
25. Peanuts	50. Papaya

Four Star Foods ★★★★

Here's a list of 50 foods that are rated 4 stars in the Star Rating System, indicating that they are super healthy for individuals managing Type 2 Diabetes:

1. Leafy greens
2. Broccoli
3. Brussels sprouts
4. Cauliflower
5. Bell peppers
6. Tomatoes
7. Avocado
8. Berries blueberries, strawberries, raspberries)
9. Cherries
10. Walnuts
11. Almonds
12. Chia seeds
13. Dark Chocolate (70 %)
14. Fatty fish
15. Tofu
16. Eggs
17. Greek yogurt (plain, non-fat)
18. Cottage cheese (low-fat)
19. Quinoa
20. Lentils
21. Chickpeas
22. Brown rice
23. Whole-grain oats
24. Lean Beef
25. Butternut squash
26. Olive oil
27. Green tea
28. Stevia Liquid Drops
29. Garlic
30. Ginger
31. Turmeric
32. Cinnamon
33. Lean poultry
34. Legumes (e.g., black beans, kidney beans)
35. Hummus
36. Green beans
37. Asparagus
38. Mushrooms
39. Artichokes
40. Greek feta cheese
41. Low-fat cottage cheese
42. Non-fat Greek yogurt
43. Milk
44. Coffee
45. Quinoa pasta
46. Seaweed (e.g., nori)
47. Green apples
48. Black Berries
49. Grapefruit
50. Lemon Water

Utilizing the Star Rating System for Meal Planning:

Congratulations on navigating our Star Rating System, a practical tool designed to simplify your food choices and support your journey in managing Type 2 Diabetes. Now, let's delve into practical examples of how to leverage this chart to create balanced and nourishing meals

Crafting a Balanced Plate:
Example Meal 1: ★★★
Lean Pork (3 stars) + Quinoa (3 stars) + Roasted vegetables (3 stars)
This meal combines lean protein, whole grains, and colorful vegetables, offering a balanced and 3-star rated plate.

Mindful Carbohydrate Choices:
Example Meal 2: ★★★★
Salmon (4 stars) + Brown rice (4 stars) + Steamed broccoli (4 stars)
Focusing on low-glycemic carbohydrates like brown rice complements the nutrient-dense salmon and vegetables, creating a balanced and 4-star rated meal.

Snacking with Purpose:
Example Snack 1 ★★★★
Greek yogurt (plain, non-fat - 4 stars) + Berries (4 stars) + Almonds (4 stars)
This snack combines protein-rich Greek yogurt with fiber-packed berries and healthy fats from almonds, offering a satisfying and 4-star rated snack.

Embracing Healthy Fats:

Example Meal 3: ★★★★

Avocado (4 stars) + Grilled tofu (3 stars) + Quinoa pasta (4 stars)
Integrating heart-healthy avocado, plant-based protein from
tofu, and nutrient-dense quinoa pasta results in a flavorful and 4-
star rated meal.

Diversifying Your Plate:

Example Meal 4: ★★★

Lentil soup (3 stars) + Mixed green salad (4 stars) + Whole-grain
roll (3 stars)
This meal incorporates legumes, leafy greens, and whole grains,
showcasing a diverse and 4-star rated plate.

Hydration Choices:

Example Beverage: ★★★★

Green tea (4 stars) + Infused water with citrus slices
Opting for beverages like green tea supports hydration with
added antioxidants, contributing to overall health.

Treating Yourself Mindfully

Example Dessert   ★★★

Fresh fruit salad (3 stars) with a drizzle of honey (2 stars)
 A dessert featuring fresh fruits and a touch of honey can satisfy
your sweet tooth while maintaining a mindful approach to sugar
intake.

Moderation is Key:Enjoy a variety of foods in moderation to create a well-rounded and enjoyable eating experience. Personalize Your Choices: Adapt the examples based on your preferences, dietary needs, and cultural considerations. Consultation with Professionals: Always consult with healthcare professionals or dietitians to tailor these examples to your specific health conditions.

Empower yourself with the Star Rating System to make informed choices, create delicious meals, and embark on a journey of nourishment that aligns with your goals in managing Type 2 Diabetes.

As we conclude our exploration into the value of food in managing Type 2 Diabetes, it becomes evident that our dietary choices play a pivotal role in shaping our health and well-being. The Star Rating System introduced in this chapter serves as a practical guide, empowering you to make informed decisions about the foods you consume.

In recognizing the impact of different foods on blood sugar levels, we've laid the foundation for a balanced and nourishing approach to nutrition. From the 1-star cautionary foods to the 4-star super healthy options, the spectrum allows for flexibility, mindful choices, and the creation of meals that not only support blood sugar control but also contribute to overall health.

As you move forward, consider the following key takeaways:

Diversity Matters: Embrace a diverse range of foods to ensure a broad spectrum of nutrients. Incorporating various food groups adds richness to your diet and supports overall health.

Balanced Plates Foster Stability: Crafting meals with a balance of macronutrients, portion control, and nutrient-dense choices promotes stable blood sugar levels and sustained energy throughout the day.

Mindful Snacking: Snacking can be an integral part of your day. Opt for nutrient-rich snacks that align with your goals, such as Greek yogurt with berries or a handful of almonds.

Flexibility and Enjoyment: Healthy eating doesn't mean sacrificing enjoyment. Treat yourself mindfully, savoring flavors, and finding joy in the nourishment you provide your body.

Consult with Professionals: Individual dietary needs vary, and it's crucial to consult with healthcare professionals or dietitians for personalized advice tailored to your specific health conditions and requirements.

But what about all the foods I love? It's challenging to steer clear of the culinary delights that have brought comfort throughout a lifetime. Our natural inclination is towards the familiar, the foods that have been a source of joy. Yet, the foods categorized here as 1-star rated might align with some of your deepest cravings. The human body is a complex interplay of intricate checks and balances.

While these foods may offer momentary satisfaction, they demand energy and effort from our body systems, disrupting the delicate balance crucial to our health. Our body, unlike the robust engine of an automobile, is a more intricate and sensitive system. We wouldn't contemplate putting the wrong oil in the engine or filling the tank with the wrong fuel.

Avoiding these 1-star foods requires dedication and effort. It's not an easy or swift process. Consider filtering your choices outside the body rather than burdening your body as the filter. When you embark on your shopping journey, prioritize items with 3 and 4 stars at the top of your list. Most importantly, shift your focus to the foods that genuinely nourish your body system."

As you embark on this journey, remember that food is not just fuel; it is a source of nourishment, pleasure, and vitality. Chapter 2 sets the stage for the chapters to come, where we will continue exploring lifestyle elements that contribute to the holistic management of Type 2 Diabetes. From exercise to sunlight, breath work to mental health, each chapter is a building block in empowering you to lead a fulfilling and balanced life with Type 2 Diabetes. So, let's continue this journey together towards a healthier, happier you.

Chapter Three

The Importance of Exercise
Introduction to Physical Activity

Living with Type 2 Diabetes demands a holistic approach, and one of the cornerstones of this approach is regular physical activity. This section delves into the vital role that exercise plays in managing Type 2 Diabetes, emphasizing its significance as a proactive and empowering measure for overall well-being.

In the journey of managing Type 2 Diabetes, exercise emerges as a powerful ally. Its importance extends beyond the confines of weight management; it is a catalyst for a cascade of positive effects throughout the body. Exercise is not merely a routine; it is a commitment to nurturing your body and enhancing its resilience.

Acknowledging the vital role of exercise is the first step toward cultivating a lifestyle that aligns with your health goals. Regular physical activity has been shown to contribute to improved insulin sensitivity, better blood sugar control, and enhanced cardiovascular health. It acts as a natural regulator, fostering a harmonious interplay within the intricate systems of your body.

As we explore the various dimensions of exercise in this chapter, remember that it is not a one-size-fits-all endeavor. Your journey towards incorporating exercise into your routine is a personal one, and the rewards are as individualized as the effort you invest. So, let's embark on this exploration of physical activity, recognizing it not only as a necessity but as a source of empowerment on your path to managing Type 2 Diabetes.

Understanding the Benefits Beyond Blood Sugar Control:

While the role of exercise in blood sugar control is pivotal, its impact reverberates far beyond, touching various facets of your overall health. In this section, we unravel the comprehensive benefits that regular physical activity brings, creating a ripple effect that extends to cardiovascular health, weight management, and even your mood.

Cardiovascular Health:
Engaging in regular exercise becomes a steadfast companion in nurturing a healthy cardiovascular system. As your heart strengthens, it pumps blood more efficiently, enhancing circulation and reducing the risk of heart-related complications. Exercise contributes to lower blood pressure and improved cholesterol levels, fostering the well-being of your heart and vessels.

Weight Management:
Exercise operates as a dynamic force in the realm of weight management. Beyond its role in burning calories, it stimulates metabolic activity, supporting your body in maintaining a healthy weight. By combining exercise with a balanced diet, you create a synergy that not only aids in weight loss but also establishes sustainable habits for long-term well-being.

Mood Enhancement:
The benefits of exercise extend to the realm of mental health, acting as a potent mood enhancer. Physical activity triggers the release of endorphins, commonly known as "feel-good" hormones, fostering a positive mental state. It provides an outlet for stress, anxiety, and tension, contributing to a balanced and resilient emotional well-being.

Understanding these multifaceted benefits unveils the holistic impact of exercise on your health. Beyond being a tool for blood sugar management, it becomes a cornerstone for building a robust cardiovascular system, maintaining a healthy weight, and cultivating a positive mindset. As you embark on your exercise journey, let these broader health benefits serve as additional motivation on your path to comprehensive well-being.

Emphasizing the Accessibility of Stretching:
In the realm of physical activity, accessibility is key, and stretching exercises emerge as an inclusive and approachable gateway to fitness. This section highlights the simplicity and universal accessibility of stretching exercises, making them an ideal starting point for individuals of all fitness levels.

The Universality of Stretching:
Stretching exercises stand out as a universally embraced form of physical activity. Regardless of age, fitness background, or health condition, stretching can be tailored to meet individual needs. Its simplicity lies in the fact that it doesn't demand advanced coordination or equipment, making it an exercise accessible to all.

Inclusivity for All Fitness Levels:
One of the remarkable aspects of stretching is its inclusivity.
Whether you're a seasoned athlete or taking your first steps into
a fitness routine, stretching exercises can be adapted to
accommodate various fitness levels. From gentle stretches for
beginners to more advanced routines for those seeking a
challenge, the spectrum is broad, ensuring that everyone can
find a suitable starting point.

Minimal Requirements, Maximum Impact:
Unlike some forms of exercise that may necessitate specialized
gear or dedicated spaces, stretching requires minimal
equipment. A comfortable and open space, combined with a
commitment to the exercises, is all that's needed. This simplicity
enhances its accessibility, making it feasible to incorporate
stretching into daily life without major disruptions.

Tailoring to Individual Needs:
Stretching is inherently flexible, allowing individuals to tailor their
routine based on their unique requirements. Whether it's
addressing specific muscle groups, improving flexibility, or
simply promoting relaxation, stretching exercises can be
personalized to align with individual fitness goals.

Emphasizing the accessibility of stretching is an invitation for everyone to partake in the benefits of physical activity. It's a reminder that, irrespective of your starting point, stretching provides a gentle and inclusive introduction to the world of exercise. As we delve into specific stretching routines later in this chapter, keep in mind the adaptable nature of stretching – an exercise accessible to all, fostering a sense of inclusivity in the pursuit of a healthier lifestyle.

In the next few pages you will find 10 basic stretches that cover various muscle groups and promote flexibility. Remember to perform each stretch slowly and gently, holding each position for about 15-30 seconds.

1. Neck Stretch:

- Gently use your hand to Slowly tilt your head to one side, bringing your ear toward your shoulder.

- Hold the stretch, feeling a gentle stretch along the side of your neck.

- Repeat on the other side.

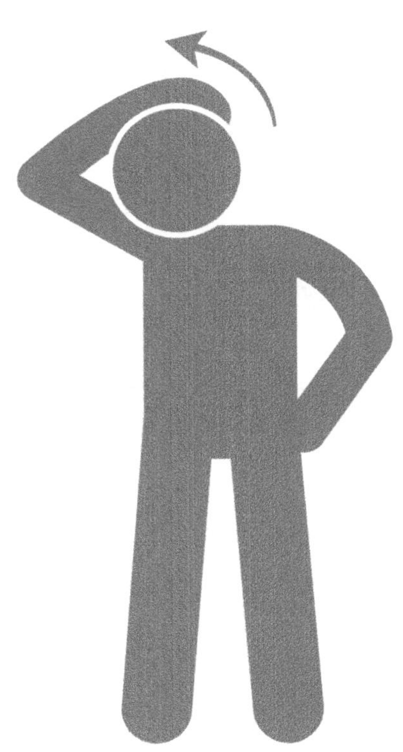

2. Shoulder Stretch:
   - Bring your right arm across your chest.
   - Use your left hand to gently pull your right arm closer to your chest.
   - Hold the stretch, feeling a gentle pull across your shoulder.
   - Repeat on the other side.

3. Triceps Stretch:

   - Raise your right arm overhead and bend your elbow, reaching your hand down your back.

   - Use your left hand to gently push on your right elbow.

   - Hold the stretch, feeling a stretch along the back of your arm.

   - Repeat on the other side.

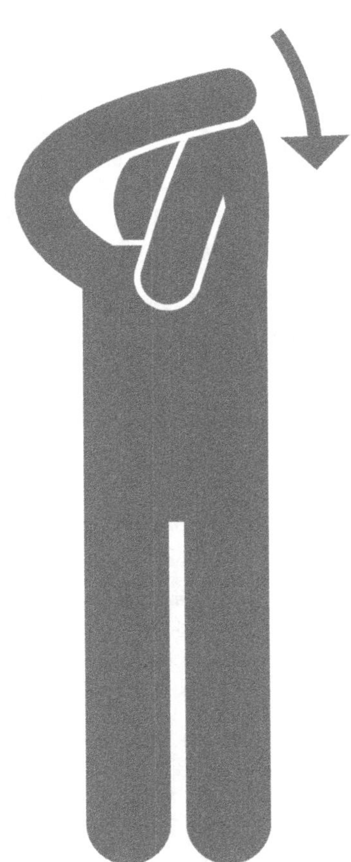

4. Chest Opener:

   - Clasp your hands behind your back.
   - Straighten your arms and lift them slightly, opening your chest.
   - Hold the stretch, feeling a gentle pull across your chest.

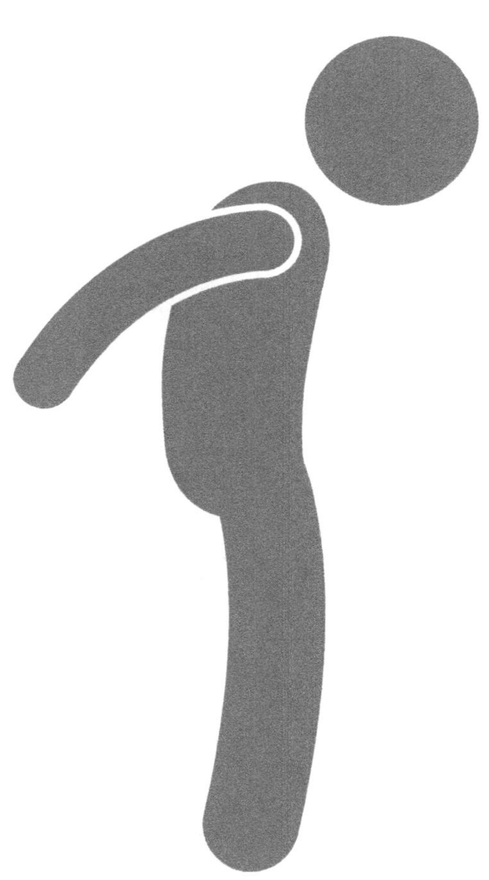

5. Back Stretch
 - Lay on your stomach face forward
place your forearms down on the floor beside your chest .
  -Use your arms to lift your chest off the floor , slightly arching
your back.
 slowly Alternate arching up and down stretching your spine.

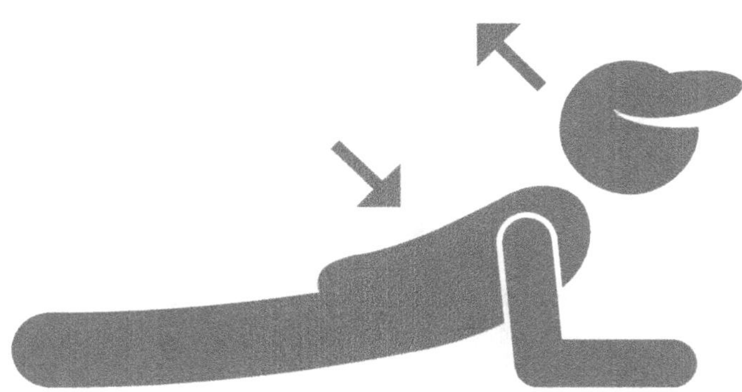

6. Seated Forward Bend:

   - Sit with your legs stretched in front of you.

   - Hinge at your hips and reach toward your toes.

   - Hold the stretch, feeling a gentle stretch along your hamstrings and lower back.

7. Full Body Stretch:

   - Stand tall, Clasp your hands over your head, Reach toward the ceiling and flip palms of hands toward the ceiling.

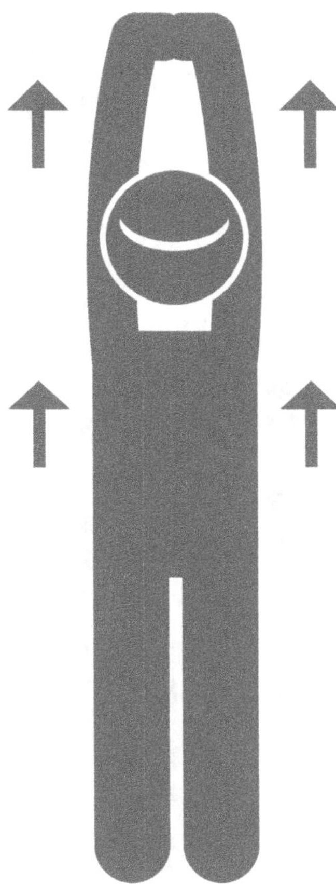

8. Quad Stretch:

   - Stand on your right leg and bend your left knee, bringing your heel toward your buttocks.

   - Hold your left ankle with your left hand, feeling a stretch in your quadriceps.

   - Hold the stretch, then switch sides.

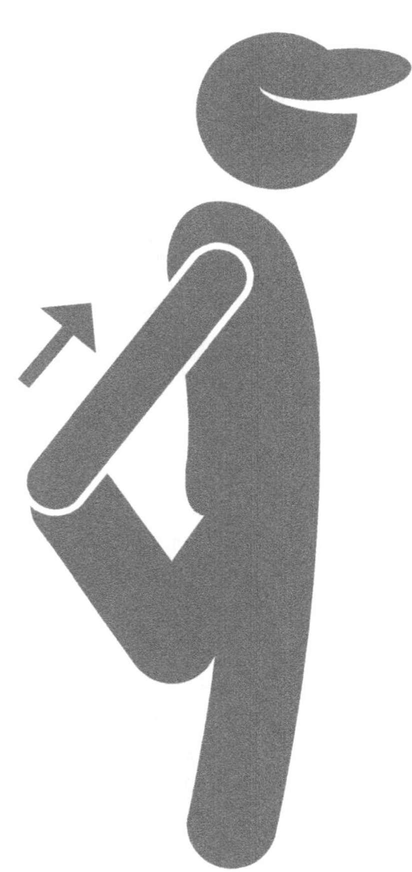

8. Ham String Stretch:

   -lay on a flat surface with legs straight. Bend the right leg and hold the thigh just under the knee. Gently pull toward the stomach. Alternate legs.

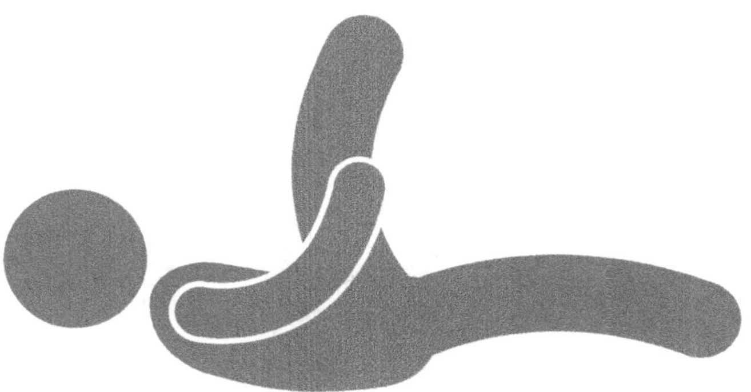

9. SideStretch:

  - Stand with arms above your head straight in the air. Lean to one side and alternate.

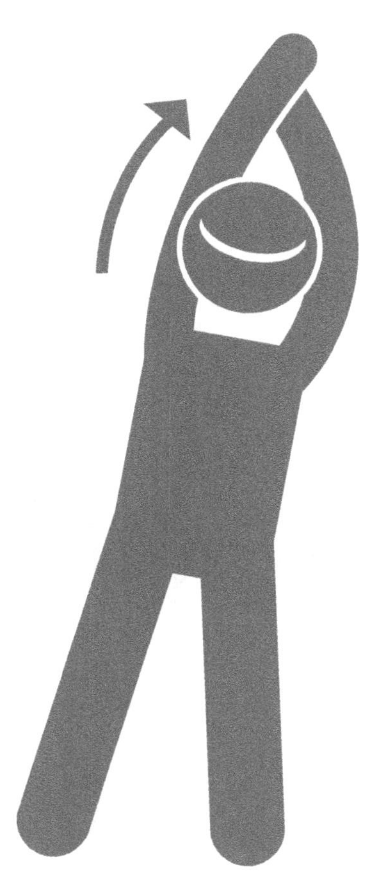

10. Calf Stretch:

   - Stand facing a wall with your hands on it.
   - Step your right foot back, keeping it straight, and press your heel into the floor.
   - Hold the stretch, feeling a gentle stretch in your right calf.
   - Repeat on the other side.

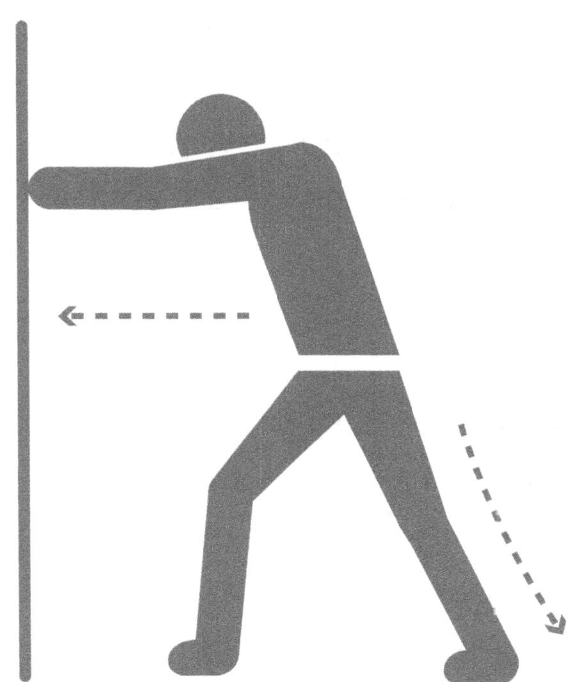

The Value of Walking:

In the expansive realm of physical activity, few exercises embody accessibility and effectiveness as seamlessly as walking. This section unravels the myriad benefits of walking, positioning it as a low-impact yet profoundly impactful form of exercise that transcends age, fitness levels, and lifestyle constraints.

The Universality of Walking:
Walking, a fundamental and instinctive human activity, is a form of exercise that resonates universally. It requires no specialized skills or equipment, making it an inclusive practice accessible to individuals of all ages and fitness backgrounds. Regardless of where you are on your fitness journey, the simple act of putting one foot in front of the other can be a transformative step toward better health.

Gentle on Joints, Mighty in Impact:
One of the distinctive features of walking is its low-impact nature. Unlike high-intensity exercises that may place stress on joints, walking provides a gentle yet effective cardiovascular workout. This makes it particularly suitable for those with joint concerns or individuals seeking a sustainable exercise routine that can be woven seamlessly into daily life.

Cardiovascular Benefits:
Walking holds the power to fortify your cardiovascular system. As you engage in brisk walking, your heart rate increases, promoting better blood circulation and oxygenation throughout the body. This, contributes to a healthier heart, and improved overall cardiovascular fitness.

Weight Management and Beyond:
Beyond its cardiovascular perks, walking plays a significant role in weight management. Whether as part of a weight loss journey or weight maintenance strategy, brisk walking aids in burning calories and maintaining a healthy body weight. Moreover, it complements dietary efforts, creating a harmonious synergy in your pursuit of a balanced lifestyle.

Mental Well-Being and Stress Reduction:
The benefits of walking extend beyond the physical realm, reaching into the domain of mental well-being. The rhythmic motion of walking, coupled with exposure to nature if done outdoors, can have a calming effect on the mind. It serves as an opportunity for introspection, stress reduction, and the release of feel-good endorphins.

Building Consistent Habits:
What sets walking apart is its adaptability to diverse lifestyles. Whether you choose to walk around your neighborhood, incorporate it into your daily commute, or embark on purposeful walking sessions, it accommodates the ebb and flow of life. This adaptability fosters the creation of consistent habits, laying the foundation for sustainable health practices.

As we unveil the value of walking, recognize it not only as an exercise but as a journey—a journey toward holistic health that begins with a simple step forward. Whether you stride through bustling streets, serene parks, or quiet corridors, each step contributes to the tapestry of your well-being, embodying the essence of simplicity, accessibility, and lasting impact.

Embarking on a walking journey requires not only the desire to move but also a structured plan that eases you into the rhythm of regular physical activity. This section proposes a beginner-friendly walking plan, designed to accommodate various fitness levels and encourage a gradual progression in intensity.

Weeks 1-2: Establishing the Foundation
Goal: Aim for 15-20 minutes of brisk walking, 3 days a week.
Begin with a comfortable pace, ensuring you can easily hold a conversation while walking.
Gradually increase your walking duration within the 15-20 minute range.
Focus on consistent, enjoyable walks to establish the habit.

Weeks 3-4: Expanding Duration
Goal: Extend your walks to 25-30 minutes, maintaining 3 days a week.
Introduce small intervals of increased pace during your walks, alternating between brisk and moderate speed.
Pay attention to your body's response and adjust the intensity based on your comfort level.
Aim for a total of 5,000 to 6,000 steps per day.

Weeks 5-6: Enhancing Frequency
Goal: Increase frequency to 4 days a week, maintaining 25-30 minute walks.
Incorporate a mix of flat and slightly inclined surfaces into your walking route.
Gradually introduce gentle inclines to enhance cardiovascular benefits.
Focus on maintaining a steady pace throughout the walk.

Weeks 7-8: Progressive Duration and Intensity

Goal: Extend walks to 35-40 minutes, with 4 days a week of walking.

Incorporate short bursts of brisk walking followed by a moderate pace.

Experiment with walking routes that include varied terrains.

Strive for 7,000 to 8,000 steps per day.

Weeks 9-10: Achieving Consistency

Goal: Maintain 4 days a week of walking, gradually increasing duration to 45 minutes.

Focus on achieving a consistent pace throughout your entire walk.

Incorporate at least one day of interval walking, alternating between brisk and moderate speeds. Aim for 8,000 to 10,000 steps per day.

Note:

- Pay attention to your body's signals and adjust the plan based on your comfort and capability.
- Stay hydrated and wear comfortable shoes.
- **Consult with healthcare professionals before beginning any new exercise routine, especially if you have pre-existing health conditions.**

This simple walking plan provides a structured approach, allowing you to gradually build endurance and intensity. Remember that progress is personal, and the goal is to foster a sustainable habit of regular walking that contributes to your overall well-being.

Exploring Exercise Options:

In today's dynamic landscape of fitness, a wealth of options awaits those seeking diverse avenues for exercise. This section navigates the realm of virtual exercise resources, shedding light on the plethora of online exercise videos and platforms that bring the gym experience directly to your home.

The Digital Fitness Revolution

In a world where technology connects us across vast distances, it also opens doors to a virtual realm of fitness possibilities. The advent of online exercise videos and platforms has transformed the way we approach physical activity, making fitness accessible from the comfort of home. Here, we explore the digital landscape that brings the gym, the yoga studio, and various workout classes to your fingertips.

Abundance of Options:

The online fitness sphere is teeming with diversity. From high-energy cardio workouts to serene yoga sessions, there's a virtual class catering to every fitness preference. Whether you're a beginner or an advanced enthusiast, the abundance of options ensures that there's a suitable workout waiting for you.

Flexibility in Scheduling:

One of the advantages of virtual exercise resources is the flexibility they offer in scheduling. No need to adhere to fixed class times; you have the freedom to choose when and where you engage in your fitness routine. This flexibility accommodates diverse lifestyles, allowing you to tailor your workouts to fit seamlessly into your daily schedule.

Access to Expert Guidance:
Online platforms often feature certified fitness instructors and experts, bringing their expertise directly to your living room. You can follow along with guided workouts led by professionals, ensuring that you receive proper guidance on form, technique, and overall fitness principles.

Comfort and Privacy:
For many, the prospect of exercising in the privacy of their own home is appealing. Virtual exercise resources provide a comfortable space where you can focus on your workout without external distractions. This setting fosters a sense of privacy, encouraging individuals who may be hesitant to engage in traditional gym settings.

Variety for Every Preference:
Whether you prefer dance-based workouts, strength training, mindfulness practices, or a combination of these, the virtual fitness realm caters to a spectrum of preferences. The diversity of classes ensures that you can explore different styles and find what resonates best with your fitness goals and interests.

As we delve into the world of virtual exercise resources, consider it not just as a substitute for traditional methods but as a vibrant addition to your fitness toolkit. The convenience, variety, and accessibility make these digital avenues a compelling option for individuals seeking a personalized and adaptable approach to their fitness journey.

Joining Exercise Groups:
In the realm of fitness, the camaraderie and shared energy of exercise groups emerge as a powerful motivator and enhancer of the overall experience. This section explores the positive impact of participating in exercise groups at gyms, parks, or community centers, highlighting the benefits of communal physical activity.

Strength in Numbers:
Embarking on a fitness journey need not be a solitary endeavor. Joining exercise groups taps into the collective strength of a community, transforming the act of physical activity into a shared and uplifting experience.

Motivation Boost:
Exercise groups serve as motivational hubs, inspiring individuals to push beyond personal boundaries. The energy of a group, the encouragement from fellow participants, and the shared commitment to health create a dynamic atmosphere that fuels motivation and propels everyone toward their fitness goals.

Structured and Varied Workouts:
Being part of an exercise group often means access to structured and varied workout routines. Trained instructors or group leaders guide participants through well-designed sessions, incorporating diverse exercises that cater to different fitness levels. This variety keeps workouts engaging and ensures a holistic approach to physical well-being.

Accountability and Consistency:
The sense of accountability within a group setting is a potent force. Knowing that others are expecting your presence fosters a commitment to regular attendance. This accountability, coupled with the social aspect of exercise groups, promotes consistency in your fitness routine.

Social Connection and Friendship:
Exercise groups transcend the physical benefits; they also nurture social connections and foster friendships. The shared experience of working toward common goals creates a sense of camaraderie. Friendships formed within these groups often extend beyond the exercise setting, providing a supportive network for overall well-being.

Adaptability to Various Fitness Levels:
Exercise groups are inclusive, accommodating participants with varying fitness levels. Whether you're a beginner or an experienced enthusiast, the group setting allows for modifications and adjustments to suit individual capabilities. This adaptability ensures that everyone can participate and progress at their own pace.

Enhanced Mental Well-Being:
The positive impact of exercise groups extends to mental well-being. The social interaction, encouragement, and shared accomplishments contribute to a positive mindset. Engaging in physical activity within a supportive community can alleviate stress, enhance mood, and create a holistic sense of well-being.

As we explore the potential of exercise groups, consider it not just as a setting for physical activity but as a vibrant community where health is cultivated collectively. Whether in the structured environment of a gym or the open spaces of a park, the shared journey toward better health becomes a celebration of unity, resilience, and the boundless possibilities that arise when individuals come together for a common purpose.

Beyond Walking: Diversifying Physical Activities:
Embracing a well-rounded approach to physical activity involves venturing beyond walking and exploring a spectrum of exercises that cater to diverse interests and fitness levels. In this section, we delve into the realm of engaging in sports, unraveling the array of activities available, each offering a unique blend of fitness, enjoyment, and community.

Engaging in Sports:
Sports activities provide an avenue for physical fitness that extends far beyond the confines of routine exercises. Whether you're seeking the thrill of competition, the joy of teamwork, or a dynamic way to stay active, exploring various sports can add a dynamic and enjoyable dimension to your fitness journey.

Tennis:
Embrace the court with a game of tennis. Suitable for all skill levels, tennis offers cardiovascular benefits, improves agility, and provides an enjoyable way to engage in physical activity. Tennis can be adapted to different intensities, making it an inclusive choice for individuals of varying fitness levels.

Golf:

Step onto the green with a round of golf. Known for its leisurely pace, golf offers a low-impact workout combined with the pleasure of being outdoors. The swinging motion engages various muscle groups, contributing to flexibility and balance. Golf's social aspect also makes it a delightful way to spend time with others.

Basketball:

For those seeking dynamic team sports, basketball is an excellent choice. Whether played casually or competitively, basketball enhances cardiovascular fitness, agility, and coordination. Engaging in a game of basketball fosters teamwork and camaraderie, making it a holistic experience beyond the physical benefits.

Swimming:

Dive into the pool for the full-body workout that swimming provides. Suitable for individuals of all ages, swimming improves cardiovascular health, builds muscular strength, and enhances flexibility. The buoyancy of water reduces impact on joints, making it an ideal choice for those with joint concerns.

Soccer:

Join the world's most popular sport with a game of soccer. Soccer combines aerobic and anaerobic elements, contributing to cardiovascular fitness and endurance. The dynamic nature of soccer engages multiple muscle groups and hones coordination skills. Additionally, the social and team elements add an extra layer of enjoyment.

Cycling:

Hit the trails or the streets with cycling. Whether on a stationary bike or riding outdoors, cycling is a low-impact exercise that improves cardiovascular health and leg strength. It offers the freedom to explore scenic routes and can be adapted to various fitness levels and preferences.

Disc Golf:

"I've personally discovered immense joy in the activity of Disc Golf. Its popularity is steadily increasing. What makes it particularly appealing is its affordability – most disc golf courses are located in public parks and offer free play. The equipment required is inexpensive, and the game is accessible to players of all ages and levels, from beginners to professionals. The courses themselves vary in difficulty, providing a diverse range of challenges.

Engaging in Disc Golf is not only a physical activity but also a social experience. Groups of all ages come together to play, and there's a strong sense of community and support fostered on social media pages dedicated to the sport. What adds to its charm is the simplicity of the game – it's enjoyable right from the very first throw, making it an accessible and entertaining activity for everyone."

As we venture beyond walking into the diverse world of sports, consider it not just as a form of exercise but as a celebration of movement, enjoyment, and the vast array of possibilities that sports bring to the realm of physical well-being.

Connecting Exercise to Blood Sugar Control:
In the intricate dance of physiology, exercise emerges as a powerful partner in the regulation of blood sugar levels. Understanding the physiological impact of exercise on lowering blood sugar unveils a crucial aspect of holistic health.

Physiological Impact:
When you engage in physical activity, your muscles demand energy. To meet this demand, your body increases its uptake of glucose from the bloodstream. Simultaneously, exercise enhances insulin sensitivity, allowing your cells to more efficiently absorb and utilize glucose. This dynamic interplay between muscles, glucose, and insulin forms the foundation of exercise's impact on blood sugar control.

Aerobic Exercise and Glucose Regulation:
Aerobic exercises, such as brisk walking, running, or cycling, induce a sustained increase in heart rate and breathing. This type of exercise has been shown to be particularly effective in improving blood sugar control. As you engage in aerobic activities, your muscles utilize glucose for energy, contributing to the reduction of blood sugar levels.

Resistance Training and Glucose Uptake:
Resistance or strength training, involving activities like weightlifting, also plays a significant role. These exercises promote muscle growth and enhance insulin sensitivity, leading to improved glucose uptake by muscles. The effects extend beyond the exercise session, contributing to more stable blood sugar levels over time.

Post-Exercise Glucose Management:
The benefits of exercise extend beyond the workout itself. After completing a session, your body continues to utilize glucose for recovery and replenishment. This ongoing glucose utilization contributes to a sustained reduction in blood sugar levels, especially when exercise is incorporated into a regular routine.

Stressing the Importance of Consistency:
In the realm of exercise and blood sugar control, consistency emerges as the linchpin for reaping sustained benefits. Emphasizing the need for a consistent exercise routine underscores the enduring impact it can have on your overall well-being.

Sustained Insulin Sensitivity:
Consistent exercise helps maintain and improve insulin sensitivity over time. Regular physical activity signals to your body that efficient glucose utilization is a continuous requirement. This sustained sensitivity ensures that your cells remain responsive to insulin, contributing to stable blood sugar levels.

Stable Blood Sugar Patterns:
The body thrives on routine. Establishing a consistent exercise routine creates predictable patterns of glucose utilization and insulin response. This predictability aids in stabilizing blood sugar levels, reducing the likelihood of sharp fluctuations that can occur in the absence of regular physical activity

Long-Term Health Benefits:
The cumulative impact of consistent exercise extends beyond immediate blood sugar control. It contributes to long-term health benefits, including reduced risk of cardiovascular issues, weight management, and overall improved metabolic health. Recognizing exercise as a lifelong commitment underscores its role as a cornerstone in the foundation of your health journey.

As you weave exercise into your lifestyle, consider it not merely as a sporadic activity but as a steadfast companion in the ongoing quest for blood sugar control and holistic well-being. The consistency of your efforts will pave the way for enduring health benefits and a harmonious relationship between your body and the intricate dance of glucose regulation.

Tailoring Exercise to Individual Preferences:

In the symphony of physical activity, the key to sustained engagement lies in the harmony between exercise and individual enjoyment. Encouraging readers to discover activities they genuinely relish paves the way for making exercise an enduring and fulfilling part of their lifestyle.

Discovering Joy in Movement:
Exercise need not be a chore; it can be a celebration of movement that brings joy. Encourage readers to explore a variety of activities, from dancing and hiking to sports and yoga, until they discover the ones that resonate with their personal preferences. When exercise becomes a source of enjoyment, it seamlessly integrates into daily life.

Building a Sustainable Routine:
The sustainability of an exercise routine hinges on its alignment with individual preferences. Whether it's the thrill of team sports, the serenity of solo walks, or the rhythm of dance, finding activities that resonate ensures that exercise is not a temporary obligation but a sustainable, lifelong commitment.

Adapting to Changing Tastes:
Preferences evolve, and so can exercise routines. Encourage readers to stay open to trying new activities and adapting their fitness regimen as their interests shift. This flexibility ensures that exercise remains an exciting and dynamic aspect of their lifestyle.

Consulting with Healthcare Professionals:
In the pursuit of personalized and health-conscious exercise, the guidance of healthcare professionals stands as a valuable compass. Emphasize the importance of consulting with healthcare professionals to craft exercise plans tailored to individual needs.

Personalized Assessment:
Healthcare professionals can conduct personalized assessments, taking into account an individual's health history, current fitness level, and any specific health concerns. This personalized approach forms the foundation for creating exercise plans that align with both health goals and medical considerations.

Addressing Health Concerns:
Individuals with specific health conditions may benefit from tailored exercise guidance. Consulting healthcare professionals ensures that exercise plans are designed to address and accommodate any health concerns, promoting a safe and effective fitness journey.

Setting Realistic Goals:
Healthcare professionals assist in setting realistic and achievable fitness goals. Whether the aim is improved cardiovascular health, weight management, or specific rehabilitation needs, having professional guidance ensures that goals are attainable and align with overall health objectives.

Monitoring Progress:
Regular check-ins with healthcare professionals allow for the monitoring of progress and adjustments to exercise plans as needed. This ongoing collaboration ensures that exercise remains a positive and health-enhancing component of an individual's routine.

Exercise is not a one-size-fits-all endeavor but as a personalized exploration guided by individual preferences and professional expertise. By tailoring exercise to personal enjoyment and consulting healthcare professionals for personalized guidance, individuals can embark on a fitness journey that aligns seamlessly with their unique needs, fostering a lifelong commitment to health and well-being.

As we draw the curtain on our exploration of the importance of exercise in managing Type 2 Diabetes, it becomes evident that physical activity is not merely a routine but a profound investment in one's overall well-being. In the intricate dance of glucose regulation, exercise emerges as a key partner, influencing not just blood sugar levels but also cardiovascular health, mental well-being, and the holistic harmony of the body.

Exercise is a transformative force, not only in the physiological realm but also in the tapestry of emotions and experiences. Whether it's the rhythmic cadence of walking, the spirited camaraderie of team sports, or the tranquil embrace of yoga, each form of movement contributes to a symphony of health, resilience, and joy.

Amidst the myriad options and diverse activities, the thread that weaves through the fabric of exercise is consistency. It is the anchor that grounds the benefits of physical activity, fostering sustained improvements in blood sugar control, insulin sensitivity, and overall fitness. The routine becomes a ritual, and the ritual becomes a source of enduring well-being.

In the chapters ahead, we will explore various facets of a lifestyle that harmonizes with the rhythms of managing Type 2 Diabetes. From the nourishment found in food to the embrace of sunlight and the melody of breath, each aspect contributes to the holistic score of health. Just as a symphony is composed of diverse instruments, your health journey is composed of multifaceted elements, with exercise being a central melody.

As you reflect on the significance of exercise, consider it not as a prescription but as an invitation to embark on a unique journey. Tailor your exercise routine to the activities that bring you joy and consult with healthcare professionals to compose a plan that harmonizes with your health goals. In the chapters that follow, we will continue to unravel the layers of a lifestyle that resonates with your well-being, empowering you to take charge and compose a life that dances to the rhythm of health.

The journey toward optimal health is a symphony, and exercise is a melody that reverberates through the chapters of your life. As we move forward, let the rhythm of movement be your guide, and may each step, stretch, and beat of your heart resonate with the vitality that fuels a life well-lived.

Chapter Four

Sunlight and Fresh Water

In the symphony of life, sunlight and fresh water emerge as the elemental duet, playing an indispensable role in sustaining the delicate balance within every living organism.

Imagine sunlight as nature's radiant gift, providing energy like a warm embrace. This energy, in the form of light, serves as a vital catalyst for various processes within our bodies:

Sunlight triggers the creation of vitamin D in our skin, a nutrient crucial for bone health and overall well-being. The natural rhythm of day and night influenced by sunlight helps regulate our internal clock, impacting sleep patterns, hormonal balance, and overall body functions. Sunlight fuels the production of energy within our cells, acting like a gentle conductor orchestrating the dance of life.

Now, picture fresh water as the fluid conductor, ensuring a seamless flow of nourishment and balance throughout the body. Water is the essence of life, keeping our cells hydrated and supporting the transportation of nutrients. It's like the conductor's baton, maintaining the flow that sustains life's melody. Just as water regulates temperature, our bodies remain in a harmonious balance, much like a perfect note in a melody. Water acts as the conductor guiding the removal of waste, ensuring a clean and clear passage for life's continuous rhythm. Together, sunlight and fresh water form an inseparable duo, nurturing life's intricate balance. Sunlight and water join forces to maintain harmony at the cellular level, ensuring the smooth functioning of processes that keep us alive and thriving. From the smallest cell to the grand orchestration of organs, sunlight and water contribute to the overall health of our bodies. They play key roles in cardiovascular health, hormonal balance, and the orchestration of bodily functions.

In simple terms, these elemental forces act as the nurturing essence, supporting life's delicate dance. Sunlight provides the energy that sparks life's processes, while fresh water ensures a smooth and flowing rhythm, sustaining the intricate balance that allows every living organism to flourish in nature's symphony.

Guidelines for Safe Sunlight Exposure: Balancing Wellness and Protection

Embracing sunlight can be beneficial for overall well-being, but it's essential to do so responsibly. Here are guidelines to ensure safe sunlight exposure, considering factors such as time of day, duration, and skin protection:

Choose the Right Time

Opt for sunlight exposure during early morning or late afternoon when the sun's rays are less intense.
Avoid prolonged exposure during peak sunlight hours (10 a.m. to 4 p.m.) when UV radiation is strongest.

Mind the Duration:

Begin with short exposure durations, gradually increasing as your skin adapts.
Aim for 10-30 minutes of sunlight two to three times a week for adequate vitamin D synthesis. Adjust based on your skin type, location, and weather conditions.

Be Mindful of Skin Type:

Fairer skin is more susceptible to sunburn. Limit exposure and use protective measures if you have lighter skin.
Individuals with darker skin may require longer exposure for sufficient vitamin D synthesis but should still practice sun safety.

Protective Clothing:

Wear loose, long-sleeved clothing and a wide-brimmed hat to shield your skin from direct sunlight.

Consider UV-protective clothing if spending extended periods outdoors.

Apply Sunscreen:
Use a broad-spectrum sunscreen with at least SPF 30 on exposed skin.
Reapply sunscreen every two hours, or more frequently if swimming or sweating.
Always check a small spot on your arm before using a new lotion.

Eye Protection:
Wear sunglasses that block both UVA and UVB rays to protect your eyes from sun damage.

Seek Shade:
Take breaks in shaded areas, especially if you're exposed to sunlight for an extended period.

Stay Hydrated:
Sun exposure can lead to dehydration. Ensure you stay well-hydrated, especially in warmer climates.

Integrating Sunlight into Daily Activities:

Morning Walks:
Start your day with a brisk morning walk, combining exercise with gentle sunlight exposure.

Gardening:
Engage in gardening activities during the cooler hours of the morning or late afternoon.

Outdoor Workouts:

Move your exercise routine outdoors, choosing shaded areas or cooler times of the day.

Lunch Breaks:

Take short breaks during lunchtime to enjoy sunlight while having a meal.

Commute Choices:

If possible, choose walking or cycling for short commutes, incorporating sunlight exposure into your daily routine.

Mindful Breaks:

Incorporate short breaks during work or study hours to step outside and soak in some sunlight.

Remember, moderation is key. These guidelines help strike a balance between reaping the benefits of sunlight and safeguarding your skin from potential harm. Always prioritize your safety and adapt these suggestions based on your personal health, location, and individual needs.

Practical Tips for Healthy Hydration Habits: Nourishing Your Body with Fluid Balance

Ensuring proper hydration is vital for overall health and well-being. Here are practical tips to establish healthy hydration habits, emphasizing the importance of adequate water intake, diverse hydration sources, and strategies for maintaining hydration throughout the day:

Set Hydration Goals:
Aim for a daily water intake based on individual needs, considering factors like age, weight, activity level, and climate. A common guideline is to consume around 8 cups (64 ounces) of water per day, but individual requirements may vary.

Carry a Water Bottle:
Keep a reusable water bottle with you throughout the day for easy access to hydration.
 Having a visible reminder encourages regular sips, ensuring consistent water intake.

Infuse Your Water:
Enhance the flavor of water by infusing it with fruits, herbs, or cucumber slices. This adds a refreshing twist without added sugars or calories.

Schedule Hydration Breaks:
Integrate short hydration breaks into your daily routine, especially if you have a sedentary job. Set reminders to take a sip every hour.

Drink Water Before Meals:
Develop a habit of drinking a glass of water before meals. Not only does this contribute to hydration, but it may also help with appetite control.

Opt for Hydrating Foods:
Include water-rich foods in your diet, such as watermelon, cucumber, oranges, and celery. These contribute to overall fluid intake.

Monitor Urine Color:
Pay attention to the color of your urine. Light yellow or pale straw color indicates proper hydration, while darker urine may signal dehydration.

Hydrate During Exercise:
Drink water before, during, and after physical activity to replace fluids lost through sweat.
Consider sports drinks for intense or prolonged exercise to replenish electrolytes.

Set Technology Reminders:
Utilize smartphone apps or smartwatches to set reminders for regular water intake. This can be especially helpful for those with busy schedules.

Explore Hydration Alternatives:
Include hydrating beverages beyond water, such as herbal teas, coconut water, and diluted fruit juices. However, be mindful of added sugars in certain beverages.

Create Hydration Stations:
Place water dispensers or pitchers in common areas at home or work to encourage family members or colleagues to hydrate regularly.

Listen to Thirst Cues:
Pay attention to your body's signals. Thirst is a natural indicator that it's time to hydrate, so listen to what your body is telling you.

Choose Hydration-Friendly Snacks:
Snack on water-rich foods like berries, cucumber slices, or yogurt to boost fluid intake between meals.

Remember that maintaining hydration is an ongoing process, and individual needs vary. Adjust these tips based on your lifestyle, activity level, and personal preferences to create a sustainable and enjoyable hydration routine that supports your overall health.

As we conclude our exploration into the symbiotic dance of sunlight and fresh water, we find ourselves immersed in the profound connection between these elemental forces and the intricate balance they bring to the canvas of life.

Sunlight, the radiant orchestrator, and freshwater, the fluid conductor, join forces to create a symphony of vitality within every living organism. From the microcosm of cells to the macrocosm of organs, their harmonious interplay sustains the delicate balance that defines optimal health.

In unraveling the chapters of this elemental journey, we've witnessed the benefits bestowed upon cardiovascular health, cellular nourishment, and the holistic well-being of both body and mind. Sunlight, with its energizing rays, breathes life into cellular processes, while fresh water flows like the rhythm that sustains the dance of existence.

Guided by the gentle light of the sun and the nurturing flow of water, we've explored the importance of safe sunlight exposure, understanding the delicate balance of time, duration, and skin protection. Practical tips have been shared to help integrate sunlight into daily activities, fostering a balanced routine that nurtures the body and soul.

As we've delved into the realm of hydration, we've embraced the significance of water as the elixir of life. Practical strategies have been unveiled to establish healthy hydration habits, encouraging diverse sources beyond water and weaving hydration seamlessly into the fabric of daily living. In concluding this chapter, let us heed the call to embrace the gifts that nature, in its wisdom, has bestowed upon us. Sunlight and fresh water stand as timeless allies, inviting us to step into the rhythm of life and bask in the vitality they offer.

As we move forward, let the symphony of sunlight and the gentle flow of water be our companions on the journey to vibrant health. May their dance inspire us to tread lightly on this Earth, cherishing the elements that sustain life's delicate balance. The chapters ahead beckon us to explore the realms of oxygen, breathwork, mental well-being, and the culmination of a holistic approach to managing Type 2 Diabetes. The dance continues, and with each step, we find ourselves closer to the harmony that nature intends for us.

Chapter Five

Breathwork - Nourishing the Essence of Life

In the grand symphony of existence, where each note resonates with the rhythm of life, the element of oxygen emerges as the invisible conductor orchestrating the dance of vitality within every living being. In this chapter, we delve into the fundamental importance of oxygen, the breath of life, and the profound connection it shares with our overall well-being.

The Breath of Life:
Oxygen, the silent maestro, is the very essence that sustains the dance of life. With each inhalation, we draw in this vital force, fueling the intricate processes within our bodies. The exchange of oxygen and carbon dioxide, a dance performed tirelessly within the lungs, forms the heartbeat of our existence. It is not merely a biological transaction but a sacred rhythm that echoes the essence of our connection to the world.

Oxygen and Cellular Symphony:
At the cellular level, oxygen orchestrates a symphony of energy production, influencing every aspect of our being. Cells, like eager musicians, respond to the life-giving cues of oxygen, harmonizing to create the melody of optimal functioning. From the beating heart to the firing neurons, oxygen is the unseen composer, weaving threads of life into the fabric of our physiological tapestry.

Breath as a Gateway to Well-being:
Beyond its physiological role, the act of breathing becomes a gateway to well-being. In the ebb and flow of breath, lies a sacred dance that transcends the mundane. Conscious breathing is an art – a mindful exploration that not only fills our lungs but touches the core of our mental and emotional realms. The intricate connection between breath and overall well-being becomes a pathway to balance, resilience, and profound self-awareness.

Embarking on a Breathwork Journey:
As we embark on this exploration of breathwork, envision it not merely as inhaling and exhaling air but as a pilgrimage into the sanctuary of life's breath. The practices that unfold in the chapters ahead invite you to embrace the transformative potential of intentional breathing. It is an invitation to dance with the rhythm of your breath, allowing it to guide you towards a state of harmony – a place where the symphony of oxygen and breath converges with the melody of your well-being.

Join us in this journey into the essence of life, where breath becomes a sacred dance, and oxygen, the silent companion, sustains the melody of existence. Together, let us unravel the tapestry of breathwork and discover the profound connections it holds for managing Type 2 Diabetes and fostering holistic health.

The Physiology of Breathing: Unveiling the Dance Within

In the intricate ballet of life, the physiology of breathing emerges as a graceful choreography, where every movement orchestrates the exchange of vital forces. Let us unravel this exquisite dance, exploring the mechanics of breathing, understanding the pivotal role of the diaphragm, and delving into the profound exchange of oxygen and carbon dioxide that sustains the symphony of our existence.

The Diaphragm: Our Respiratory Maestro:

At the heart of the respiratory dance is the diaphragm, a remarkable muscle nestled beneath our lungs. As the principal conductor of this rhythmic symphony, the diaphragm orchestrates inhalation and exhalation with exquisite precision. During inhalation, the diaphragm contracts and flattens, creating a vacuum that draws air into the lungs. Upon exhalation, the diaphragm relaxes, allowing the lungs to expel air. This elegant interplay of muscle and breath forms the cornerstone of respiratory mechanics.

Inhalation: A Symphony of Oxygen:

As the diaphragm descends, the chest cavity expands, inviting air to rush in through the nostrils or mouth. This inhaled air carries with it the life-giving oxygen, an essential fuel for cellular function. The intricate network of bronchial tubes and alveoli within the lungs acts as the stage for this exchange, allowing oxygen to journey into the bloodstream.

Exhalation: The Dance of Release:
Upon completing its journey through the bloodstream, oxygen finds itself in the cells, supporting energy production and sustaining life's myriad processes. Simultaneously, the cellular dance produces carbon dioxide, a byproduct that must gracefully exit the stage. Exhalation becomes the vehicle for this release, allowing carbon dioxide to journey back through the bloodstream to be expelled from the body.

The Dance Beyond the Lungs:
The physiological impact of conscious breathing extends far beyond the lungs. Conscious, intentional breath influences the autonomic nervous system, regulating heart rate, blood pressure, and stress responses. By engaging in mindful breathing, we invoke the parasympathetic nervous system, fostering a state of calm and balance.

Influence on Cellular Processes:
Conscious breathing becomes a guiding force in the delicate ballet of cellular processes. By providing an optimal environment for oxygen exchange, intentional breathwork supports cellular respiration, energy production, and the maintenance of overall cellular health. This, in turn, reverberates through the entire organism, influencing organ systems, cognitive function, and emotional well-being.

The Breath: A Bridge to Presence:
As we unravel the physiological intricacies of breathing, we uncover the profound connection between conscious breath and our holistic well-being. Breath becomes more than a mere biological function; it becomes a bridge to presence, a pathway to balance, and a rhythmic dance that sustains the symphony of life.

In the chapters ahead, let us continue this exploration, deepening our understanding of breath's influence on mental, emotional, and physical realms. Together, we shall embrace the transformative potential of conscious breathing on the journey to managing Type 2 Diabetes and fostering vibrant health.

Benefits of Oxygen to the Body and Cells: Nourishing Every Corner of Life

Let's take a simple stroll into the world of oxygen and how it becomes the superhero for every little cell in your body. Imagine oxygen as tiny helpers that bring energy and life to every part of you.

The Marvelous Journey of Oxygen:

So, here's the cool part – when you breathe in, your body gets a visit from these superhero oxygen molecules. They hitch a ride through your nose or mouth, making their way into your lungs. Now, your lungs are like a busy city with tiny streets called bronchial tubes, and they guide the oxygen molecules to their destination.

Oxygen's VIP Treatment in Cells:

Once in your lungs, oxygen hops onto a red blood cell for a VIP ride through your bloodstream. These cells travel to every nook and cranny of your body, delivering oxygen to the cells that need it. It's like a special delivery service, ensuring that each cell gets the energy it needs to do its job.

Cellular Joy with Oxygen:

Now, here's where the magic happens. In your cells, oxygen joins a fantastic party called cellular respiration. It's like a mini power plant inside each cell, where oxygen helps turn food into energy. This energy keeps everything running smoothly – your heart beating, your muscles moving, and your brain buzzing with ideas.

Carbon Dioxide's Exit Dance:
As the cells use oxygen, they throw a little party themselves and create a byproduct called carbon dioxide. Don't worry; this isn't a troublemaker. Carbon dioxide joins the journey back through your bloodstream, and when you exhale, it says goodbye to the outside world. It's like a graceful dance of exit – in and out, in perfect harmony.

The Big Picture – Happy Body, Happy You:
So, why is all this oxygen and cell talk important? Well, when your cells are happy and energized, your entire body feels amazing. You have the energy to play, think, move, and be your awesome self. It's like giving your body the best fuel it needs to run smoothly – and that's the superhero power of oxygen!

As we continue this adventure, we'll explore how your breath can be a superpower, influencing your mood, stress levels, and even helping manage Type 2 Diabetes. So, keep breathing, and let the oxygen superheroes do their fantastic work in your incredible body!

Consequences of Diminished Oxygen: A Look at What Happens When Oxygen Takes a Break

Let's chat about what happens when our superhero, oxygen, takes a little break. Imagine oxygen as your body's best friend, and when it's not around enough, things get a bit wonky.

When Oxygen Takes a Breather:
So, oxygen is usually the life of the party, making sure everyone's happy and energetic. But sometimes, if we're not breathing well or something's not quite right, oxygen might not show up in the right amounts.

Feeling a Bit Tired:
Imagine your cells waiting for their friend oxygen to arrive, but it's fashionably late. Your body might start feeling a bit tired because the cells aren't getting the energy they need. It's like trying to run a race without your favorite sneakers – not as fun.

Brain Fog and Forgetfulness:
Now, your brain loves oxygen, and when it doesn't get enough, it might start feeling a bit foggy. You know that feeling when you can't remember where you put your favorite toy? That's what happens when oxygen isn't there to give your brain a high-five.

Not So Happy Organs:
Oxygen is like a superhero for your organs, keeping them healthy and happy. But if it takes a break, your organs might not work as well. It's like a little grumble from your tummy or a not-so-happy dance from your heart.

The Oxygen Comeback Plan:
The good news is, we can always bring oxygen back to the party! Taking nice, deep breaths, getting fresh air, and moving our bodies all help oxygen feel welcome again. It's like giving a warm welcome to your superhero friend, saying, "Hey, we missed you!"

Introduction to Breathwork Practices: Breathing Exercises for a Happy Body

Now that we've chatted about our superhero oxygen and how important it is, let's dive into something fun – breathing exercises! It's like giving your body a little workout for happiness. Ready? Let's explore!

Breathwork - What's That?:

Breathwork is like a special menu of exercises just for your breath. It's not about running a marathon; it's about giving your lungs a little love and making sure oxygen gets a front-row seat in your body.

Deep Belly Breaths: The Happy Belly Workout:

Ever tried filling your belly with air like a balloon? That's a deep belly breath! Breathe in slowly, letting your belly expand like you're filling it with the yummiest air. Then exhale slowly, feeling your belly go back down. It's a happy workout for your belly and a chill pill for your body.

Balloon Breaths – Inflate and Deflate:

Imagine you're blowing up a balloon. Breathe in slowly, imagining your lungs filling up the balloon. Then, exhale like you're letting all the air out. It's a playful way to keep your lungs feeling fresh and happy.

4-7-8 Breathing – The Relaxation Secret:
This one's a bit magical! Inhale quietly through your nose for four counts, hold your breath for seven counts, and exhale slowly through your mouth for eight counts. It's like a secret code that tells your body it's time to relax. Try it whenever you need a little calm.

Breathwork Playtime:
Breathwork is like a playdate for your breath. You can do it sitting, standing, or even lying down – anywhere you feel comfy. The more you practice, the more your body will thank you with good vibes.

Why Do Breathwork?:
Breathwork isn't just for fun; it's like giving your body a super boost. It helps with stress, makes your brain feel happy, and keeps your superhero oxygen doing its dance. Plus, it's a cool way to manage Type 2 Diabetes like a superhero manager!

So, give these breathwork exercises a try, and let the good vibes roll. We're on this breathy adventure together, unlocking the secrets of managing Type 2 Diabetes with a smile. Keep breathing, and let the happy body party begin!

The Magic of Meditation: A Calming Adventure for Your Mind
We're about to embark on a magical adventure – the world of
meditation. It's like giving your mind a cozy blanket and a warm
cup of cocoa. Ready to discover the wonders of calm? Let's dive
in!

Meditation – What's That?:
Meditation is like a little vacation for your mind. It's not about
doing tricks or sitting in a weird pose; it's simply about finding a
comfy spot and letting your mind relax.

Mindful Breathing – Hello, Calmness:
Sit or lie down comfortably. Close your eyes and take a deep
breath. As you breathe in, think, "I'm breathing in." As you
breathe out, think, "I'm breathing out." It's like a gentle
reminder to your mind to chill and enjoy the breath.

Body Scan – Checking In with Yourself:
Imagine a warm light scanning your body from head to toe. As it
moves, notice how each part feels. It's like giving your body a
little high-five and saying, "Hey, I'm here for you." This helps
relax both your mind and body.

Nature Visualization – A Mental Getaway:
Close your eyes and picture a beautiful place in nature. It could
be a beach, a forest, or a meadow. Imagine the sights, sounds,
and smells. It's like taking your mind on a mini-vacation without
leaving your comfy spot.

Loving-Kindness Meditation – Sending Good Vibes:
Think of someone you care about – a friend, family member, or even yourself. In your mind, say, "May you be happy, may you be healthy, may you be safe, may you be at ease." It's like spreading good vibes and warmth to the people you love.

Meditation Playtime:
Meditation isn't a serious business; it's your mind's playtime. You can do it for a few minutes or longer – whatever feels right. The more you practice, the more your mind will appreciate the calm moments.

Why Meditate?:
Meditation is like giving your mind a spa day. It helps with stress, boosts your mood, and brings a sense of calm. Plus, it's a fantastic tool for managing Type 2 Diabetes like a peaceful superhero.

So, find a comfy spot, let your mind unwind, and enjoy this magical journey of meditation. We're on this calm adventure together, discovering the wonders of a peaceful mind. Keep meditating, and let the magic unfold!

Embracing Art Therapy: Unleashing Creativity for a Happy Mind

We're about to dive into the colorful world of art therapy. It's like giving your mind a canvas to play on, and the best part? You don't need to be an artist – just a sprinkle of imagination. Ready to explore the magic of creativity? Let's jump in!

Art Therapy – What's the Buzz?:

Art therapy is like a creative hug for your mind. It's not about creating a masterpiece; it's about expressing yourself and letting your imagination run free. You can do it with colors, shapes, or even doodles – it's your personal playground.

Coloring Books – A Magical Canvas:

Ever tried coloring in a book? It's not just for kids; it's a fantastic way to relax. Grab your favorite coloring book and let your creativity flow. The best part? No rules, just fun! The author of this book has even created some cool coloring books in different themes – nature, mandalas, and more!

Coloring Your Way to Calm:

Pick a coloring page that speaks to you. Maybe it's a serene landscape or a whimsical mandala. As you color, let your mind wander and enjoy the soothing dance of colors. It's like a mini-vacation for your imagination.

Expressive Doodling – Scribble Away Stress:
Doodling isn't just for the margins of your notebook; it's a mindful way to let go of stress. Grab a piece of paper and let your pen dance freely. Your mind guides the way, and before you know it, you've created a unique piece of art.

Art Playtime:
Art therapy is your personal playtime. You don't need fancy materials – just what makes you happy. Whether it's crayons, markers, or even digital tools, let your creativity shine. The goal isn't perfection; it's the joy of creating.

Why Art Therapy?:
Art therapy is like a burst of sunshine for your mind. It helps reduce stress, boosts your mood, and taps into your inner artist. Plus, it's a delightful tool for managing Type 2 Diabetes with a dash of creativity.

So, grab your colors, embrace the joy of art, and let your imagination run wild. We're on this colorful adventure together, exploring the magic of creativity. Keep creating, and let the artful journey unfold!

As we wrap up our exploration into the realms of breath, meditation, and the vibrant canvas of art therapy, let's take a moment to savor the essence of what we've uncovered. Chapter 5 has been a journey into the holistic well-being of mind and body, embracing practices that go beyond the physical to touch the realms of tranquility and creativity.

A Symphony of Breath:
We began by unraveling the wonders of breath – the dance of oxygen that sustains life. From the physiological ballet within our lungs to the magic of conscious breathing, we discovered the profound impact of breath on our overall well-being. Through simple breathwork exercises, we opened the door to a realm where every inhale and exhale becomes a step towards calmness.

Meditation's Calming Embrace:
The journey continued into the serene landscapes of meditation – a tranquil escape for the mind. From mindful breathing to nature visualizations, we delved into practices that offer moments of stillness in the midst of life's hustle. Meditation became a gentle companion, guiding us towards inner peace and a sanctuary of calmness.

Art Therapy's Expressive Canvas:
The chapter unfolded further into the expressive world of art therapy, where colors and creativity became our allies. Whether through the therapeutic strokes of coloring books or the freeform dance of expressive doodling, we tapped into the joy of creation. Art therapy emerged as a pathway to self-expression and a delightful tool for cultivating harmony.

A Tapestry of Holistic Well-being:
As we conclude this chapter, let's recognize that true well-being extends beyond physical health. It encompasses the symphony of breath, the calmness of meditation, and the vibrant colors of creativity. These practices are not just tools for managing Type 2 Diabetes; they are threads woven into the tapestry of a harmonious life.

So, dear reader, take a moment to appreciate the breath that sustains you, the calmness that envelops you, and the creativity that flows through you. In the chapters ahead, we'll continue this exploration, weaving a narrative that intertwines practical insights, mindful practices, and the artistry of well-being. Until then, breathe, meditate, create, and let the harmony unfold.

Conclusion

Closing the Chapter on Type 2 Diabetes

As we reach the final pages of this book, it's time to reflect on the key discoveries that have unfolded in our exploration of managing Type 2 Diabetes. Let's take a moment to revisit the gems that now reside in your knowledge treasure chest.

The Symphony of Well-being:
We began by understanding the essence of Type 2 Diabetes, peeling back the layers to explore its impact on the body. From the basics of insulin resistance to the potential effects on organs, we unveiled the importance of early detection and diagnosis.

Navigating Nutrition's Landscape:
Chapter 2 became a compass in the world of food, emphasizing the profound role nutrition plays in managing Type 2 Diabetes. From the power of a healthy diet to the star-rated guide, we crafted a roadmap for making food choices that nourish both body and soul.

Mind-Body Harmony Unleashed:
Chapters 3 to 5 transported us into the realms of exercise, sunlight, fresh water, breathwork, and mental well-being. We danced through the benefits of stretching, walked into the embrace of sunlight and fresh air, discovered the magic of oxygen, and embraced the calming arts of meditation and creativity.

A Wholesome Tapestry:
In our collective journey, we stitched together a wholesome tapestry that extends beyond the physical aspects of health. It's a tapestry woven with the threads of conscious breath, tranquil meditation, and the vibrant hues of creativity.

A Grateful Farewell:
As you close this book, know that you hold a toolkit filled with insights and practices to embark on a healthy journey. The pages are now yours to revisit, each chapter a guidepost on your path to well-being.

Thank you for entrusting your time and attention to this exploration. Your commitment to understanding and managing Type 2 Diabetes is a commendable step towards a healthier you. May the wisdom gathered within these pages accompany you on your journey to a vibrant and joyful life.

Wishing you the very best on your health adventure. Until we meet again on the pages of well-being.

Here's a list of resources that can further support and enrich your journey in managing Type 2 Diabetes:

1.American Diabetes Association (ADA):
   - Website: [American Diabetes Association] (https://www.diabetes.org/)

2.Centers for Disease Control and Prevention (CDC):
   - Diabetes information: [CDC Diabetes] (https://www.cdc.gov/diabetes/index.html)

3.Mayo Clinic:
   - Diabetes information and resources: [Mayo Clinic - Diabetes] (https://www.mayoclinic.org/diseases-conditions/diabetes)

4.National Institute of Diabetes and Digestive and Kidney Diseases (NIDDK):
   - Diabetes resources: [NIDDK - Diabetes] (https://www.niddk.nih.gov/health-information/diabetes)

5. Diabetes Forecast:
   - Diabetes magazine by ADA: [Diabetes Forecast] (https://www.diabetesforecast.org/)

6. MyPlate by USDA:
   - Dietary guidelines and meal planning: [ChooseMyPlate] (https://www.choosemyplate.gov/)

7. Exercise and Physical Activity for Older Adults:
 - Tips and guidelines from the National Institute on Aging:
[Exercise and Physical Activity]
(https://www.nia.nih.gov/news/research-interactions-
blog/2019/05/exercise-and-physical-activity)

8. Mental Health America:
 - Mental health resources: [Mental Health America]
(https://www.mhanational.org/)

9. Art Therapy Coloring Books by the Author:
 - Explore the relaxing and creative world of coloring with books
by the author.

**Simple Patterns Coloring Book For Teens And Adults
ASIN: B0CRHPFDZ2**

**Coloring Book For Adults Floral Stained Glass
ASIN: B0CMB8XPQY**

**10. Diabetic Delights Large Print :101 Diabetes-Friendly
Recipes For Healthy Living: Large 8.5 by 11 inch Size
https://www.amazon.com/dp/B0CGKVFTLN**

Remember to consult with healthcare professionals for
personalized advice and guidance on managing Type 2 Diabetes.
These resources provide valuable information and support to
complement your health journey.

Notes

Notes

Notes